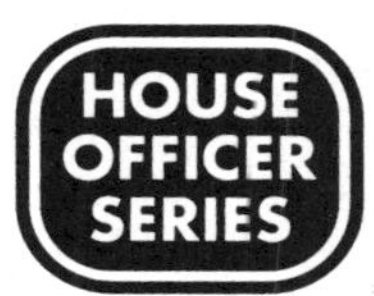

ICU Care

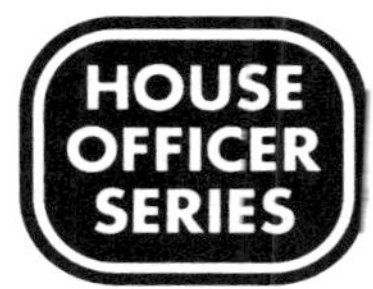

ICU Care

Mark A. Helfaer, M.D.

Director
Pediatric Intensive Care Unit
Children's Hospital of Philadelphia
Associate Professor of Anesthesia and Pediatrics
University of Pennsylvania
School of Medicine
Philadelphia, Pennsylvania

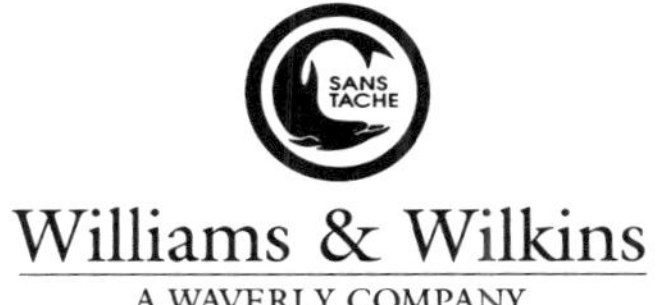

BALTIMORE • PHILADELPHIA • LONDON • PARIS • BANGKOK
BUENOS AIRES • HONG KONG • MUNICH • SYDNEY • TOKYO • WROCLAW

Editor: Charles W. Mitchell
Managing Editor: Grace E. Miller
Marketing Manager: Rebecca Himmelheber
Production Coordinator: Carol Eckhart
Project Editor: Paula C. Williams
Typesetter: Peirce Graphic Services, Inc
Printer & Binder: Vicks Lithograph & Printing

351 West Camden Street
Baltimore, Maryland 21201-2436 USA

Rose Tree Corporate Center
1400 North Providence Road
Building II, Suite 5025
Media, Pennsylvania 19063-2043 USA

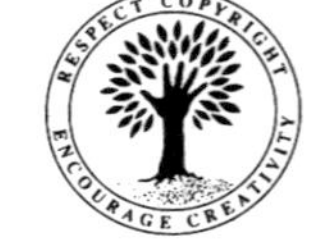

Accurate indications, adverse reactions and dosage schedules for drugs are provided in this book, but it is possible that they may change. The reader is urged to review the package information data of the manufacturers of the medications mentioned.

Printed in the United States of America

Library of Congress Cataloging-in-Publication Data

(insert catalog card here)

The publishers have made every effort to trace the copyright holders for borrowed material. If they have inadvertently overlooked any, they will be pleased to make the necessary arrangements at the first opportunity.

To purchase additional copies of this book, call our customer service department at **(800) 638–0672** or fax orders to **(800) 447–8438.** For other book services, including chapter reprints and large quantity sales, ask for the Special Sales department.

Canadian customers should call **(800) 665–1148,** or fax **(800) 665–0103.** For all other calls originating outside of the United States, please call **(410) 528–4223** or fax us at **(410) 528–8550.**

Visit Williams & Wilkins on the Internet: **http://www.wwilkins.com** or contact our customer service department at **custserv@wwilkins.com**. Williams & Wilkins customer service representatives are available from 8:30 am to 6:00 pm, EST, Monday through Friday, for telephone access.

98 99 00 01 02
1 2 3 4 5 6 7 8 9 10

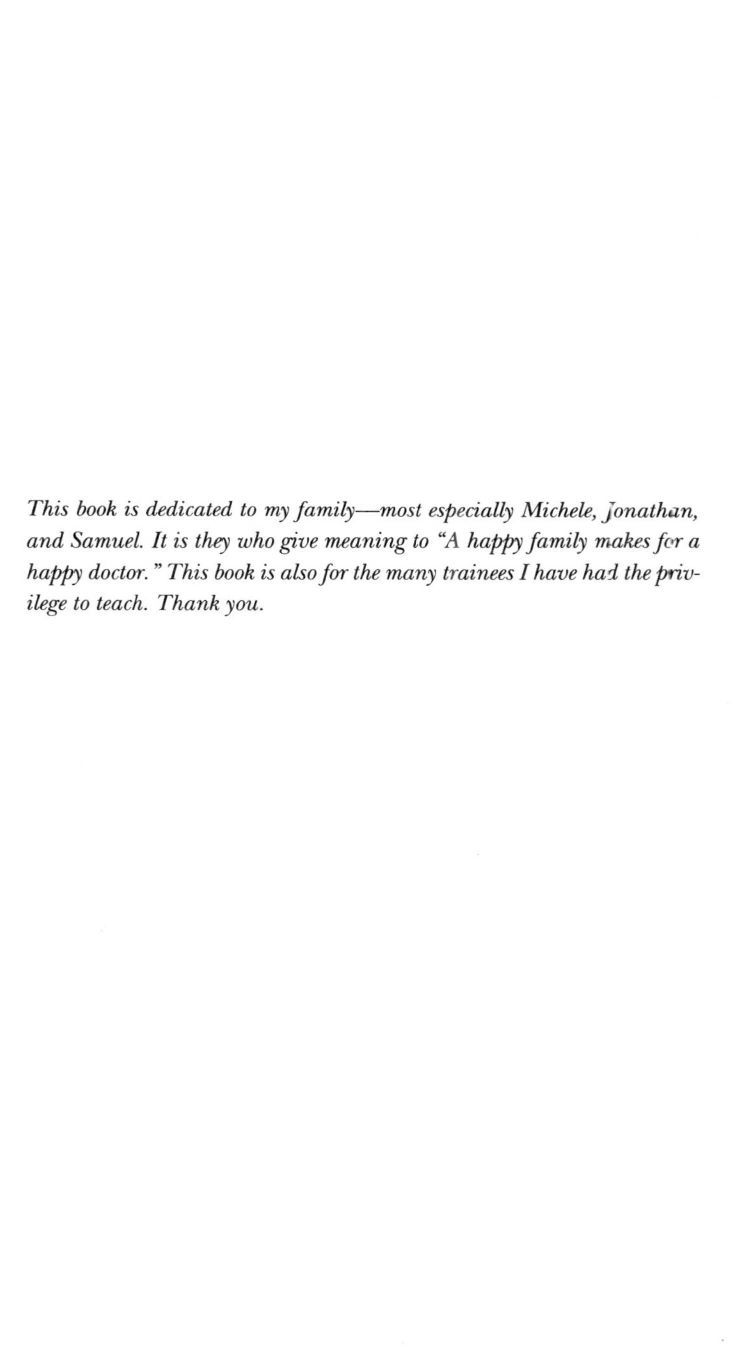

This book is dedicated to my family—most especially Michele, Jonathan, and Samuel. It is they who give meaning to "A happy family makes for a happy doctor." This book is also for the many trainees I have had the privilege to teach. Thank you.

Preface

As economic constraints more and more dictate medical practice, medicine is focused on cost-effective delivery of care. Health care practitioners in training spend more of their time learning in an outpatient setting and less time learning in the inpatient setting. This is the exact opposite of the pattern of health care training for the last 100 years. Today, health care professionals graduating from training programs are often less comfortable and less proficient with issues of inpatient care. This situation has spawned the "hospitalist" as a physician who is focused on cost-effective and high-quality inpatient care. In comparison to outpatient medicine, inpatient care is often faster paced and focused on particulars and specifics because the relative few patients admitted to inpatient units are substantially sicker compared to inpatients of even 10 years ago.

Every discipline has its guiding principles; inpatient care is no different. Its principles apply to all aspects of inpatient medicine, and specific principles are unique to individual inpatient units. These principles of inpatient management in the various areas of the hospital are the focus of this handbook. *ICU Care* is not a comprehensive text for directing the care of individual patients and units; although, many such texts exist. This book provides an overview of the approach in the different units and focuses on the priorities placed on the management of these patients. *ICU Care* serves as an introduction to issues and disease-specific priorities and serves as a primer for the dialect of inpatient medicine. It is the trainee in danger of being overwhelmed by the minutiae of inpatient management who will most benefit from this book. This book also is directed at the trainee who may be inspired to pursue a career as a hospitalist. It is for these trainees that *ICU Care* has been written. We hope that the proliferation of hospitalists will improve the care of inpatients and help other health care providers better understand inpatient medicine.

Contributors

Susan W. Aucott, M.D.
Assistant Professor
Department of Pediatrics
The Johns Hopkins University School of Medicine
Baltimore, Maryland

Anish Bhardwaj, M.D.
Assistant Professor of Neurology, Neurological Surgery and Anesthesiology/Critical Care Medicine
The Johns Hopkins University School of Medicine
Baltimore, Maryland

Clifford S. Deutschman, M.S., M.D., F.C.C.M.
Associate Professor of Anesthesia and Surgery
University of Pennsylvania School of Medicine
Philadelphia, Pennsylvania

Jeff Dodd-o, M.D., Ph.D.
Department of Anesthesiology and Critical Care Medicine
The Johns Hopkins Medical Institutions
Baltimore, Maryland

John J. Downs, M.D.
Emeritus Professor of Anesthesia and Pediatrics
The University of Pennsylvania School of Medicine
Director of Respiratory Rehabilitation Service
The Children's Hospital of Philadelphia
Department of Anesthesiology and Critical Care Medicine
Philadelphia, Pennsylvania

Rebecca D. Elon, M.D., M.P.H.
Associate Professor of Medicine
The Johns Hopkins University School of Medicine
Medical Director
The Johns Hopkins Geriatrics Center
Baltimore, Maryland

Mary Jo Fishburn, M.D.
Assistant Professor of Medicine
The Johns Hopkins University School of Medicine
Good Samaritan Hospital
Baltimore, Maryland

Mark A. Helfaer, M.D., F.C.C.M.
Director, Pediatric Intensive Care Unit
Children's Hospital of Philadelphia
Associate Professor of Anesthesia and Pediatrics
University of Pennsylvania
School of Medicine
Philadelphia, Pennsylvania

Keith C. Kocis, M.D., M.S., F.A.A.P., F.A.C.C.
Medical Director, Cardiothoracic Intensive Care Unit
Childrens Hospital, Los Angeles
Assistant Professor of Pediatrics
University of Southern California School of Medicine
Los Angeles, California

Diane C. Lipscomb, M.D.
Pediatric Intensive Care Unit
Sunrise Hospital and Medical Center
and Sunrise Children's Hospital
Las Vegas, Nevada

Daniel Nyhan, M.D.
Associate Professor
Chief, Cardiac Anesthesia
Department of Anesthesiology and Critical Care Medicine
The Johns Hopkins Medical Institutions
Baltimore, Maryland

Patricia M. Quigley, M.D.
Assistant Professor of Pediatrics
The Johns Hopkins University School of Medicine
Director of Pulmonary Services
Mt. Washington Children's Hospital
Baltimore, Maryland

Adnan I. Qureshi, M.D.
Fellow
Neuroscience Critical Care Division
The Johns Hopkins University School of Medicine
Baltimore, Maryland

Peter Rock, M.D.
Professor of Anesthesiology and Medicine
Chief, Barnes Hospital Division of Anesthesiology
Department of Anesthesiology
Washington University School of Medicine
St. Louis, Missouri

Steven P. Schulman, M.D.
Associate Professor
Department of Medicine
Director, Coronary Care Unit
The Johns Hopkins Hospital
Baltimore, Maryland

James Shear, M.D.
Assistant Professor of Anesthesiology
Department of Anesthesiology
Washington University School of Medicine
St. Louis, Missouri

John A. Ulatowski, M.D., Ph.D.
Assistant Professor of Neurology, Neurological Surgery, and Anesthesiology/Critical Care Medicine
The Johns Hopkins University School of Medicine
Baltimore, Maryland

Contents

1

Neonatal Intensive Care

Susan W. Aucott

Medical history can be essential in anticipating and evaluating many conditions in the newborn, beginning with the maternal history. Maternal age, parity, obstetric history, underlying medical problems, and family history may have direct implications for the current pregnancy. The pregnancy history itself yields insight into many issues that directly affect fetal growth and well-being. For example, maternal use of drugs, alcohol, or tobacco can have direct effect on the fetus. Insulin-Dependent Diabetes Mellitus can affect the pregnancy at many stages by increasing risk for malformations, affecting fetal growth, and increasing the risk in the newborn for multiple complications such as hypoglycemia, polycythemia, hypertrophic cardiomyopathy, and hyperbilirubinemia. The birth history also can provide information regarding risk factors for sepsis, birth injury, hypoxic–ischemic encephalopathy, respiratory distress, or apnea secondary to maternal medications.

RESUSCITATION

Most neonatal resuscitations occur in the delivery room; here, a neonate must initiate respirations and transition from a fetal circulatory pattern to a mature circulatory pattern. These efforts may be hampered by complications of the pregnancy, birth, or by medications given to the mother around the time of birth. Because of the additional complications brought on by cold stress, the infant should briefly be dried and placed on a radiant warmer before delivery room resuscitation.

AIRWAY

The first step in assuring an open airway is to place the infant supine with the neck slightly extended by placing a rolled blanket under the infants shoulders. Next, the mouth and nose should be suctioned to clear the airway of fluid and secretions. A bulb syringe provides adequate suctioning. Deep suctioning during the first few minutes after birth is not recommended because of vagally induced bradycardia. In the case of thick meconium-stained amniotic fluid, endotracheal intubation is recommended to provide clearing of the pharynx.

BREATHING

If an infant has not initiated respiration after the stimulation of drying and suctioning, resuscitation with bag and mask ventilation must be initiated. Appropriate mask size must be used to obtain an adequate seal and to avoid trauma to the infants face. Preterm infants require a #0 mask while term infants use a #1 mask. One hundred percent oxygen always should be used for resuscitation. Because a newborn's lungs are fluid filled, the initial breath may require 30 to 40 cm H_2O pressure to inflate the lungs. Subsequent breaths require 15 to 20 cm H_2O pressure at a rate of 40 to 60 breaths per minute. The exception to using bag and mask ventilation in a newborn is a prenatal diagnosis or suspicion of congenital diaphragmatic hernia. Air entry into the gastrointestinal tract from the bag and mask ventilation causes intestinal distension that will further compromise ventilation; in these infants, proceed directly to endotracheal intubation.

Frequently, infants respond to resuscitation by initiating spontaneous respiration. If ongoing ventilation is needed because of no or inadequate respirations, an endotracheal tube is recommended. Assembling the appropriate size of equipment is required, which is based on infant size. A size 0 laryngoscope blade is used in preterm infants, and a size 1 is used in full-term infants. Endotracheal tubes are based on weight, which can be anticipated by gestational age: 2.5 mm for < 1000 gm (< 28 weeks); 3.0 mm for 1000 to 2000 gm (28 to 34 weeks); 3.5 mm for 2000 to 3000 gm (34 to 38 weeks); and 3.5 to 4.0 mm for > 3000 gm (> 38 weeks). A stylet helps insert the tube. Appropriate tube position is verified by auscultation of bilateral, equal breath sounds, and observation of chest rise with ventilation.

In infants with spontaneous respirations, the need for blow by oxygen must be assessed. Underlying cardiopulmonary processes may impair adequate oxygenation, resulting in central cyanosis. If the infant responds to blow by oxygen, a persistent oxygen requirement can be assessed by slowly withdrawing the oxygen source while observing the color of the infant.

CIRCULATION

Most newborn resuscitations are resolved by establishing adequate ventilation because most of the pathophysiologic processes relate to the initiation of respirations or achieving adequate oxygenation. Further resuscitation may be required in infants who have had in utero processes that compromise cardiac function, or who have suffered acute blood loss, such as with placental previa, placental abruption, or a cord accident. These infants may have persistent bradycardia or hypoperfusion despite establishment of adequate ventilation. Chest compressions are necessary when the heart rate is below 60 or when the heart rate is 60 to 80 and not increasing despite 15 to 30 seconds of ventilation. Epinephrine can be given via the endotracheal tube (0.1 to 0.3 mL/kg of 1:10,000 solution). Further medications, particularly volume expanders, require an intravenous line placement, which easily can be placed via the umbilical vein. A 3.5 or 5.0 French umbilical catheter is inserted into the vein via the umbilical stump until the catheter tip is just past the level of the skin and blood return is present in the catheter. Volume expanders such as 5% Albumin, Normal Saline or whole blood can then be given in 10 mL/kg doses. During a prolonged resuscitation, or if a metabolic acidosis is documented, sodium bicarbonate can be given. Because of the risk of intraventricular hemorrhage associated with rapid bicarbonate infusion in preterm infants, a 4.2% (.5 mEq/mL) solution is given over at least 2 minutes, at a dose of 2 mEq/kg. Sodium bicarbonate should only be given after effective ventilation is established. In the presence of a respiratory acidosis, the administration of bicarbonate can lead to a further increase in CO_2 and thus further decrease the pH and worsen the acidosis.

APGAR SCORES

The apgar score was designed to assess the need for resuscitation in a newborn and to, subsequently, assess the effectiveness of the resuscitation. The score is based on five assessments, which include heart rate, respirations, tone, grimace, and color. Each assessment receives a score of 0 to 2, with 0 meaning absence and 2 meaning normal. A score is given at 1 minute of life and again at 5 minutes. If the 5 minute score is less than 7, additional scores should be obtained every 5 minutes up to 20 minutes or until the scores are 8 or greater. The apgar score assesses response to resuscitative efforts and documents the condition of the infant at birth, but does not delineate the cause of low scores nor does it provide a prognosis.

PHYSICAL EXAMINATION

The initial physical examination provides critical information for the care of the newborn. Assessing infant size, including birth weight, head circumference, and length, in conjunction with a gestational age assessment, such as the revised Ballard examination, gives insight into the infants condition, allows anticipation of specific complications, and can direct diagnostic evaluation. By comparing the three growth parameters to normative curves for gestational age, one can determine if the infant's size is appropriate, small (< 10th percentile), or large (> 90th percentile) for gestational age. Small for gestational age infants are at higher risk for complications such as hypothermia, hypoglycemia, and polycythemia. The underlying cause of their small size may have various implications. Infants who are symmetrically small have height, weight, and head circumference less than the 10th percentile, which could be the result of a congenital infection or an underlying genetic disorder. For those who are asymmetrically growth retarded and have more appropriate head growth, weight is most severely affected, which could represent utero placental insufficiency as a result of maternal conditions such as hypertension or preeclampsia. Large for gestational age infants are at increased risk for hypoglycemia and birth injury. The causes for infants being large for gestational age include maternal diabetes, maternal obesity, or it could be familial.

In addition to assessing growth, the physical examination in the newborn infant should focus on excluding malformations.

Recognizing patterns of malformations may help classify the infant as having a genetic disorder or syndrome, which provides important information regarding prognosis and associated problems not yet determined. Early recognition of some conditions may simplify treatment. For example, congenital hip dislocation, when diagnosed in the newborn period, can be treated by positioning with a harness. If not recognized until later in infancy, surgical correction becomes necessary.

NEUROLOGY

In both term and preterm infants, the neurologic examination and underlying neuroanatomy are developing and changing, putting neonates at risk for specific pathologic processes. The neurologic examination relies more on muscle tone and the presence of primitive reflexes such as the suck, plantar grasp, palmar grasp, and Moro reflexes. The birth process itself can place the infant at risk for specific neurologic injuries.

Periventricular–Intraventricular Hemorrhage

Cerebral vasculature in preterm infants differs from that in term infants. The germinal matrix, in the subventricular zone, has a rich arterial supply which feeds a capillary bed of large irregular vessels. These vessels are supported poorly and do not have collagen or muscle, making them more susceptible to rupture. The immature vessels are remodeled into a mature capillary bed as the germinal matrix regresses. In addition, preterm infants have perforating arteries, arising from meningeal arteries, that regress near term. These additional vessels result in a shift of the water-shed region to the periventricular region. Thus, any fluctuation of cerebral blood flow, particularly coupled with hypoxia, can result in rupture of the immature vessels, and a germinal matrix hemorrhage. Significant hemorrhage results in rupture into the lateral ventricles. Ventricular dilatation can develop when the hemorrhage is progressive. Intracerebral hemorrhage may be associated with the intraventricular hemorrhage and is most likely a result of an associated venous infarction. The risk of intraventricular hemorrhage increases with decreasing gestational age and has an overall incidence of 35 to 45%

of all infants less than 32 weeks gestation. Fifty percent of all hemorrhages occur in the first day of life, with 90% occurring by day 3. The severity of the hemorrhage can be graded by head ultrasound appearance. Grade I is a germinal matrix hemorrhage. Grade II consists of intraventricular hemorrhage of less than 50% of ventricular area. Grade III is an intraventricular hemorrhage of greater than 50% of ventricular area and dilation of the lateral ventricles. Grade IV hemorrhages include intracerebral involvement.

Clinically, in preterm infants, hemorrhage can present in three ways. A catastrophic presentation consists of a sudden onset of lethargy with a full fontanelle associated with a metabolic acidosis and anemia. A saltatory presentation consists of several intermittent episodes of decreased activity, apnea, or bradycardia. The majority of infants have a silent presentation in which no clinical correlation is noted. Because of the frequency of silent bleeds, head ultrasounds are done routinely on all preterm infants less than 32 weeks. Initial head ultrasounds are done on the third day of life, unless clinically indicated earlier, and again at approximately 1 week of life to catch the small number whose bleeds occur late, or to assess for progression of previously documented bleeds. The importance of periventrical–intraventricular bleeds lies in the complications and the effect on prognosis. Infants with Grades I and II hemorrhages do as well as other preterm infants of similar gestational ages without hemorrhage. With a Grade III hemorrhage, infants have a 40% incidence of major neurologic sequelae, whereas with a Grade IV, they have an 80% incidence. Infants with intraventricular hemorrhage are at risk for posthemorrhagic hydrocephalus with an increasing risk and increasing severity of hemorrhage. This can occur days to weeks after the initial hemorrhage. Blood in the CSF results in an arachnoiditis, resulting in failure to reabsorb the CSF and subsequent hydrocephalus. Thus, in any infant with an intraventricular hemorrhage, serial head ultrasounds should be performed to assess for progressive ventricular dilatation. Weekly head circumference measurements allow one to monitor appropriate head growth. Treatment includes serial lumbar punctures to relieve the pressure, if the ventriculomegaly becomes significant. In 50% of infants, the hydrocephalus resolves spontaneously and the remainder require ventriculo–peritoneal shunts.

The best prevention of intraventricular hemorrhage is the prevention of preterm birth. In caring for preterm infants at risk for hemorrhage, avoidance of processes that cause hypoxia, fluctuations in blood pressure, decreases in cerebral blood flow (such as hypocapnia) or sudden changes in osmolarity (such as rapid sodium bicarbonate infusion) will decrease the risk of intraventricular hemorrhage.

Periventricular Leukomalacia

Preterm infants are at increased risk for hypoxic injury in the periventricular region, because of the vascular anatomy previously described. Hypoxic injury to the region will not be apparent on head ultrasound until 2 to 4 weeks later. It may be seen as an increased echogenicity or may actually have cysts present. A head ultrasound done at 4 weeks of age helps identify infants with periventricular leukomalacia (PVL). Documenting PVL on head ultrasound indicates that the infant is at high risk for developing cerebral palsy. The injury impairs myelination for the corticospinal tracts that descend through this region.

Hypoxic–Ischemic Encephalopathy

Perinatal events place newborns at risk for hypoxia, ischemia, or both, which can lead to significant encephalopathy. Antepartum events, such as utero placental insufficiency, maternal hypotension, or hemorrhage from placenta previa, can lead to oxygen deprivation to the brain through either hypoxia or decreased perfusion. Intrapartum events, such as cord prolapse, prolonged delivery, or failure of initiation of respirations, can have similar results. Postnatal events, such as recurrent apnea, large patent ductus arteriosis, or cardiopulmonary processes producing hypoxia, can contribute to hypoxic–ischemic encephalopathy, particularly in preterm infants.

The neonatal neurologic syndrome that results from a hypoxic–ischemic insult can be divided into three groups: mild, moderate, and severe. Infants classified as mild are described as hyperalert and hyperexcitable. Although they also may have mild involvement of other organ systems documented by hematuria or elevated lever transaminases, there is no mortality or morbidity associated with this group. Those classified as moderate have hypotonia and suppressed primitive reflexes. Other organ system involvement usually is apparent. Respiratory support may be required. Mortality in the moderate group is 5%, with 21% of survivors with neurologic sequelae. Severe hypoxic–ischemic encephalopathy presents immediately with deep stupor or coma, and the infant is flaccid with absent primitive reflexes. Pupillary and oculomotor responses are intact. Periodic breathing or absent respirations are common. Seizures are common by 6 to 12 hours of life. During the second 12 hours of life, there is an increase in level of alertness, but is accompanied by more seizures and apneic spells. During the next period of 24 to 72 hours of life, stupor again occurs, often associated with respiratory arrest. Oculomotor disturbances may now become evident, and pupils may be fixed or reactive, but constricted. In preterm infants, this neurologic syndrome is commonly associated with severe intraventricular hemorrhage. Significant involvement of other organ systems, such as cardiac, renal, and hepatic, complicate the infant's course; mortality is 75%. Imaging of the head is helpful, and may show diffuse hypodensity or hemorrhages. EEGs also can indicate the severity of the insult, but are less helpful in terms of predicting outcome. Those infants who survive with the severe form of encephalopathy will show gradual improvement over days to weeks, but all will have neurologic sequelae. The sequelae include feeding difficulty as a result of poor oromotor function, initial hypotonia that can progress and cause hypertonia and cerebral palsy, and mental retardation. Other than severity of the clinical neurological syndrome, no single clinical or laboratory test can provide a prediction of the outcome. Poor prognosis is more common in those infants with seizures in the first 24 hours of life or whose seizures are difficult to control. The duration of the neonatal neurologic abnormalities is helpful. Infants whose neurologic examination returns to normal by 1 week do well, whereas those with prolonged abnormalities have more severe sequelae.

Clinical management of infants with hypoxic–ischemic encephalopathy primarily consists of supportive care. Attention to adequate oxygenation and blood pressure helps avoid any further cerebral injury. Hypoglycemia and hypocalcemia can be seen and should be treated with IV supplements. Fluid restriction is recommended in cases of cerebral edema and when there is a risk for Syndrome of Inappropriate Antidiuretic Hormone (SIADH). Control of seizures is crucial because ongoing seizure activity accelerates cerebral metabolic rate, further aggravating the hypoxic–ischemic injury.

Seizures

Seizures in the newborn infant frequently are caused by an underlying neurologic disorder. The clinical manifestations of neonatal seizures are divided into four types: subtle, tonic, clonic, and myoclonic. Subtle seizures occur in both term and preterm infants and may be associated with other seizure types. Subtle seizures movements consist of eye deviation, sucking or chewing, apnea, or extremity movements such as bicycling, swimming, or rowing. Of these movements, only the eye deviation is consistently associated with abnormal EEG activity. Other aspects of subtle seizures, though reflective of an abnormal neurologic examination, may not be associated with specific EEG activity and, as a result, may not be responsive to anticonvulsant therapy. Tonic seizures can be either generalized or focal. Generalized tonic seizures consist of tonic flexion or extension of the neck, trunk, and upper extremities, with extension of the lower extremities. This mimics the decorticate or decerebrate posturing seen in older children. This seizure type is more common in preterm infants and is not always associated with EEG changes. Focal tonic seizures are manifested by asymmetric posturing of the trunk or limbs and is consistently more associated with EEG changes.

Clonic seizures are associated most consistently with EEG activity. Clinically, they consist of rhythmic jerks, which can be focal or multi focal. Focal seizures may denote an underlying structural lesion in the contralateral cerebral hemisphere, but also can be seen in more generalized abnormalities such as hypoglycemia. Myoclonic seizures consist of rapid contractions of flexor muscles and can be focal, multifocal, or generalized. These seizures are rare in newborns, but mimic infantile spasms in older infants.

These clinical manifestations of seizures must be differentiated from other types of movements in the neonate. Both clonus and jitteriness can be confused with seizure activity. Clonus or jitteriness is caused by stimulus or position change and can be suppressed by restraint of the limb. Seizures are not stimulus-sensitive and cannot be stopped by restraint. Seizures more commonly are associated with autonomic changes.

Investigating the causes of neonatal seizures becomes important because neurologic outcome is determined by the underlying neurologic process. The most common cause of seizures in the newborn is hypoxic–ischemic encephalopathy. These seizures typically occur in the first 72 hours of life. The next most common cause of seizures in newborns is central nervous system infection. Bacterial sepsis in neonates, usually as a result of group B β-hemolytic streptococcus or Escherichia coli (E. coli), can cause meningitis. Early onset infection is seen in the first 72 hours, whereas late onset infection would present at 3 to 6 weeks of age. Other manifestations of sepsis would be present, and the infant may be irritable, obtunded, or have a full fontanelle. Viral infections also can produce meningitis or encephalitis. These tend to present slightly later than the early onset bacterial infections. A classic example is the herpes simplex virus, which can produce a hemorrhagic encephalitis with associated seizures at 5 to 7 days of life.

Any form of intracranial hemorrhage can lead to seizures. Severe periventricular–intraventricular hemorrhage in preterm infants may cause seizures. Subarachnoid hemorrhage can occur in association with asphyxia in preterm infants, but can be seen in isolation as a result of trauma in full-term infants. Infants may appear well and develop seizures on the second or third day. Diagnosis may be suspected from bloody spinal fluid on lumbar puncture, but is difficult to differentiate from a traumatic tap. Diagnosis must be confirmed by CT scan. The prognosis in isolated subarachnoid hemorrhage is excellent. Another form of hemorrhage associated with trauma is subdural hemorrhage. The history is frequently remarkable for either a precipitous delivery, forceps delivery, or a large for gestational age infant delivery. These historical events can result in excessive molding that causes tearing of superficial venous channels over the cerebral hemisphere. Clinically, the infant initially may appear well, but subsequently develops seizures, poor feeding, or vomiting and may have jaundice or anemia. A diagnosis is made by CT scan. Management depends on the clinical condition of the infant and progression of the bleed and varies from observation to surgical drainage. Cerebrovascular ischemia can occur in utero with resultant infarction. These infants present with focal or multifocal clonic seizures and may have hypotonia. These seizures may occur as isolated events, but may represent a hypercoagulable state, such as in protein S or C deficiency. Diagnosis is made by neuroimaging and there are usually long-term focal deficits.

Another neurologic abnormality that can lead to seizures is underlying CNS malformations. Malformations, such as holoprosencephaly or lissencephaly, may be associated with other congenital malformations readily apparent on examination. Other forms, such as hydranencephaly or schizencephaly, commonly are isolated malformations, and no dysmorphic features can be noted on physical examination. Neuroimaging is required to define the malformation, and prognosis is poor because of the global involvement.

Metabolic derangements can lead to seizures, with hypoglycemia and hypocalcemia being most common in neonates. Hypoglycemia typically occurs on the first day of life and is seen most commonly in infants of diabetic mothers who are hyperinsulinemic at birth. It also can be seen in large for gestational age infants, growth-retarded infants, and as a result of asphyxia or sepsis. Treatment with intravenous glucose is recommended and can be given as 10% glucose at 80 mL/kg per day, which provides 5 mg/kg per minute of glucose. This should be increased as needed to stabilize blood glucose levels over 40 mg/dL. When the hypoglycemia is severe or the infant is symptomatic, particularly with seizures, a bolus of 10% glucose at 2 mL/kg will acutely increase the serum glucose. This must be followed by the continuous infusion because a rapid increase in the serum glucose further stimulates insulin production, resulting in recurrence of the hypoglycemia. The glucose infusion then can be weaned off gradually as enteral nutrition is established. With prompt attention to the hypoglycemia, infants do well neurologically. Less commonly, hypoglycemia may be caused by an inborn error of metabolism, particularly organic acidemia and glycogen storage disease. An associated acidosis or prolonged intravenous glucose need may suggest an inborn error of metabolism.

Hypocalcemia in infants also can cause seizures. This usually results from an underlying cause, such as maternal diabetes, maternal hyperparathyroidism, DiGeorge Syndrome, or asphyxia. The hypocalcemia typically presents at 48 to 72 hours of life. Treatment consists of intravenous bolus of calcium gluconate at 100 mg/kg every 6 hours for 4 doses.

Maternal substance abuse, such as heroin and methadone, can lead to a narcotic abstinence syndrome. Infants are hyperalert and jittery and may develop diarrhea, tachypnea, and seizures. The time of presentation depends on the timing of the mother's last drug use and the drug half-life. Infants exposed to heroin present at 24 to 48 hours of life, whereas those exposed to methadone develop symptoms at 7 to 10 days of life because of the longer half-life of the drug. A standardized scoring system is available that can guide the need for treatment. With an increasing number of symptoms, and thus higher abstinence score, the risk of seizures increases. Treatment consists of phenobarbital at loading doses of 15 to 20 mg/kg and subsequent maintenance doses of 4 to 6 mg/kg. Alternatively, paregoric can be used in doses of 4 to 6 drops every 6 hours.

Because of the broad range of possible causes of seizures, the diagnostic investigation of a newborn with seizures must begin with a review of the history. Underlying maternal health, risk factors for sepsis, birth asphyxia, or trauma must be assessed. On physical examination, signs of systemic disease, such as sepsis or meningitis, any abnormalities of the neurologic examination, and presence of anomalies or dysmorphic features, must be evaluated to guide the investigation. Initial screening laboratory tests should include a complete blood count with differential blood glucose and electrolytes including calcium and magnesium, a blood gas analysis to assess oxygen and acid-base status, blood and CSF cultures, CSF analysis, and an EEG. Documented electrical seizure activity is helpful in newborns because seizures may not be clinically obvious. Further testing will be determined by the initial results, which may include neuroimaging, viral titers or cultures, or metabolic screens. Treatment begins with correcting any underlying metabolic abnormality such as hypoglycemia or hypocalcemia. Additionally, appropriate ventilation and perfusion must be secured. If seizure activity persists and is not caused by a metabolic problem, anticonvulsant therapy is initiated. Phenobarbital is given as a 20 mg/kg intravenous bolus. Additional boluses may be required to achieve a serum concentration of 40 μg/mL. If adequate phenobarbital levels are unable to control seizures, phenytoin can be given as an intravenous bolus of 20 mg/kg. In status epilepticus, the addition of short-acting benzodiazepines may control the seizures acutely. Short-acting benzodiazepines can be given intravenously at a dose of 0.05 mg/kg or as a continuous infusion at 0.1 to 0.3 mg/kg per hour until seizure control is achieved. In infants whose seizures are a result of an acute insult, the anticonvulsant medications can be weaned off with low risk of seizure recurrence. Those infants with underlying lesions or malformations require ongoing anticonvulsant therapy with serial EEGs over the first year of life to assess an appropriate time to discontinue the medications.

RESPIRATORY

The evaluation of pulmonary processes in the newborn period can be complicated by the normal physiologic transitions that must occur at the time of birth. The infant must expand fluid-filled lungs, subsequently absorb the remaining fluid, and transition from the fetal circulatory pattern to a mature circulatory pattern. Signs of respiratory difficulty in newborns include grunting, nasal flaring, intercostal retractions, tachypnea (respiratory rates greater than 60 breaths per minute), cyanosis, or apnea. Mild grunting or flaring may occur in the first hour of life in otherwise healthy infants, but should not persist or be associated with other signs of distress. When infants present with respiratory symptoms, particularly cyanosis or tachypnea, distinguishing pulmonary from cardiac pathology can be difficult. A chest radiograph showing an enlarged or irregular cardiac shadow is consistent with cardiac pathology, or the pulmonary infiltrate of pneumonia, respiratory distress syndrome, or meconium aspiration and suggests a pulmonic process. When the cause remains unclear, a hyperoxia test is indicated. The infant is placed in 100% oxygen, and an arterial blood gas is obtained. If the oxygen level is less than 100 mm Hg, significant right-to-left shunting associated with cyanotic heart disease is present. An oxygen level of greater than 150 mm Hg is consistent with a pulmonary process causing the oxygen requirement. Levels of 100 to 150 mm Hg are equivocal and cannot distinguish between pulmonary and cardiac causes.

A common reason for evidence of respiratory difficulties is underlying hypoxia. Providing oxygen frequently alleviates the symptoms. This commonly is provided to infants via a humidified oxygen hood. Oxygen content can be varied to provide the appropriate level needed. Assessment of adequate oxygenation can be accomplished noninvasively by pulse oximeter. This gives a value of the percent saturation of hemoglobin. Normal values on the first hour of life are in the low 90s and increase to the upper 90s shortly after. A transcutaneous oxygen sensor also provides a noninvasive method to assess oxygenation, but provides a correlation of paO_2. Normal values are 50 to 60 mm Hg at birth increasing to 70 to 90 mm Hg. In preterm infants, prolonged exposure to hyperoxia can contribute to the development of retinopathy of prematurity. Thus, adequate monitoring of oxygenation becomes essential, not only to avoid hypoxia, but also to prevent hyperoxia. The disadvantage of pulse oximetry is that at high saturations, large changes in paO_2 result in only small increments in the oxygen saturation, making it more difficult to assess hyperoxia. The disadvantage of transcutaneous oxygen monitoring is that it requires warming of the skin at the probe site, which in preterm infants can cause burns. Neither system allows assessment of ventilation. Repeated sampling of arterial blood can be facilitated by placing an umbilical arterial catheter. Under sterile conditions, the umbilical artery is dilated, and a catheter is advanced to the appropriate level. Correct position is verified on x-ray, with high lines at T6 to T10, and low lines at L2 to L4, to avoid placing catheters near the renal arteries. Placement of an umbilical arterial catheter has many complications that include vasospasm causing loss of perfusion to the lower extremities, clot formation resulting in hypertension, poor renal blood flow or poor blood flow to the lower extremities, and acute blood loss with disconnection or severing of the line. These risks must be weighed with the need for frequent monitoring in an acutely ill infant.

When respiratory distress persists despite providing oxygen, further support is indicated, particularly if hypoxia or hypercarbia persist. Continuous positive airway pressure (CPAP) can be provided via nasal prongs along with oxygen. Levels of 4 to 6 cm H_2O can be used, with optimal levels for individual infants varying with progression of the underlying pulmonary process. If CPAP fails to improve ventilation or oxygenation or there is inadequate respiratory effort, assisted ventilation is required. Positive pressure ventilation most commonly is used in newborns. Ventilation is produced by adjusting peak inspiratory pressure (PIP), positive end expiratory pressure (PEEP), rate, and inspiratory to expiratory time ratio. Increasing PIP increases mean airway pressure, which improves oxygenation and ventilation. Increasing PEEP also can increase mean airway pressure, but can cause increased air trapping with a resultant increase in $paCO_2$. Increasing the rate improves ventilation with minimal effect on oxygenation. Increased inspiratory time augments mean airway pressure and can improve oxygenation; however, it also can interfere with adequate exhalation and thus decrease ventilation. The disadvantage of assisted ventilation, especially over prolonged periods, is the resultant barotrauma to the lungs. High frequency ventilation is another form of assisted ventilation, which allows improved ventilation with lower mean airway pressures and thus less barotrauma.

Transient Tachypnea of the Newborn

A common cause of respiratory symptoms on the first day of life is transient tachypnea of the newborn (TTN). Delayed resorption of amniotic fluid in the lungs occurs, impeding adequate gas exchange. The infant presents with tachypnea, grunting, flaring, retractions, and hypoxia shortly after birth. The history is frequently remarkable for either cesarean section birth or precipitous vaginal delivery. The infant may have mild symptoms and require only oxygen supplementation or may have significant distress and require assisted ventilation. A chest radiograph is not specific and may be indistinguishable from the diffuse infiltrates of pneumonia. Frequently in TTN, fluid will be in the right major fissure. The distinguishing feature of TTN is that the symptoms resolve in 24 to 48 hours, and the radiograph returns to normal in the same period. Because the initial symptoms are identical to sepsis or pneumonia, infants are treated with antibiotics until documentation of negative blood cultures and normalization of the radiograph. No long-term sequelae are associated with TTN.

Respiratory Distress Syndrome

The most common cause of clinical problems in preterm infants is respiratory distress syndrome (RDS) as a result of pulmonary immaturity and lack of adequate surfactant production. RDS occurs with increasing frequency at decreasing gestational ages. Other risk factors include maternal diabetes and perinatal asphyxia. Infants present with respiratory symptoms either immediately after delivery or within 6 hours of birth, which consist of tachypnea, grunting, flaring, retracting, and cyanosis. Symptoms can progress and worsen over the first 72 hours of life before improvement starts. Chest radiograph can show a hazy, diffuse infiltrate described as a ground glass appearance with airbronchograms. In more severe cases, there can be opacification of the lung fluids with loss of the heart border. Optimally, treatment begins prenatally with administration of corticosteriods to the mother at least 24 to 48 hours before delivery, but no longer than 7 days before delivery. Prenatal corticosteriods hasten lung maturity and thus decrease the incidence of RDS. Postnatally, appropriate support of ventilation and oxygenation must be established.

Surfactant administration can decrease the severity of RDS and significantly decreases mortality. Surfactant can be given prophylactically in the delivery room as rescue therapy after documenting the presence of RDS. The disadvantage of surfactant therapy is that it requires placement of an endotracheal tube for administration and can be associated with transient hypoxia or bradycardia during administration. Prophylactic dosing can be helpful in low birth weight infants in which the incidence of RDS is very high. In infants greater than 28 weeks gestation, there is a decreasing incidence of RDS, risking unnecessary treatment of infants. Dosing regimens differ between the commercially available surfactant products, but early administration enhances the beneficial effects. In addition, there is an additive effect when both antenatal steroids and postnatal surfactant are used. Because the clinical presentation and radiographic findings of RDS are identical to that of Group B streptococcal sepsis or pneumonia, infants with clinical evidence of RDS are evaluated for sepsis and treated with antibiotics. The complications of RDS primarily relate to the need for mechanical ventilation and include pneumothorax, pulmonary interstitial emphysema, and bronchopulmonary dysplasia.

Bronchopulmonary Dysplasia

The combination of oxygen toxicity and barotrauma, particularly when imposed on premature infants, can result in neonatal chronic lung disease or bronchopulmonary dysplasia (BPD). The original description of BPD occurred after the introduction of mechanical ventilation for the treatment of preterm infants with respiratory distress syndrome. BPD is described as occurring in all patients who remain oxygen dependent at 28 days of life after mechanical ventilation and have persistent abnormalities on their chest radiograph. With the improved survival of very low birth weight infants, more infants required prolonged mechanical ventilation because of other complications of prematurity such as apnea. This has led to a significant increase in a milder form of chronic lung disease. Because of this, an alternate definition is used to attempt to describe those infants who truly have underlying lung disease, which consists of any infant with a persistent oxygen requirement at 36 weeks corrected gestational age. With either definition, chronic lung disease becomes more prevalent with decreasing birth weight. Clinically, infants require mechanical ventilation and oxygen therapy early in life usually for treatment of RDS, but may require such therapy as a result of any cause of respiratory failure. By 1 to 2 weeks of age, the infant has not shown the classic improvement of RDS, but the chest radiograph may still indicate persistent RDS. Typically, the more coarse radiographic pattern of BPD with areas of hyperinflation and areas of coarser densities appears at 3 to 4 weeks of age. Additionally, episodes of bacterial or viral sepsis in the first month of life are associated with the development of BPD. Infants with BPD require ongoing respiratory support, which includes mechanical ventilation and oxygen supplementation as needed. The administration of corticosteroids in the presence of BPD improves lung function and facilitates weaning from the ventilator, but does not change the duration of oxygen therapy. Optimal age of starting treatment, dose schedule, and length of treatment are still not clear because many different protocols are used. The short-term benefits of improved lung function must be weighed against the side effects of the steroids, which include hypertension, hyperglycemia, and poor growth. Concerns of increased risk of infection have not been born out. Fluid management becomes important in infants with chronic lung disease caused by poor pulmonary compliance predisposing them to pulmonary edema. Fluid intake should be minimized to the amount needed to provide adequate caloric intake. Diuretics frequently are used to control pulmonary edema. Providing adequate nutrition becomes a primary goal. Infants frequently have high caloric needs because of the increased work of breathing. High-caloric density formulas can provide maximal intake of calories while still restricting fluid intake. As part of the pathophysiologic response to the barotrauma, these infants have airway-smooth muscle hypertrophy and airway hyperreactivity. Inhaled β-agonists reduce airway resistance.

Mortality in infants with severe BPD is higher than that in preterm infants of similar gestational age and can be caused by respiratory failure, superimposed infection, or cor pulmonale. The majority of infants, particularly those with milder degrees of chronic lung disease and who have adequate growth and nutrition, can show gradual improvement in pulmonary function and have radiographic signs of healing. However, there is a long-term increase in airway hyperreactivity and increased neurodevelopmental impairments.

Pneumothorax

Extrapulmonary extravasation of air occurs more frequently in the neonatal period than any other time of life. Spontaneous pneumothorax occurs in approximately 1% of all live births. In addition, a pneumothorax can be the result of underlying pulmonary pathology such as pneumonia, meconium aspiration syndrome, or RDS. A pneumothorax also can be the result of barotrauma from assisted ventilation or from use of high peak inspiratory pressures during a vigorous resuscitation at birth. An infant with a pneumothorax presents with tachypnea, which may be accompanied by grunting or cyanosis. On physical examination, breath sounds are decreased over the affected side, and the cardiac apex may be shifted. Transillumination can be useful for acutely diagnosing a pneumothorax, with increased illumination of the thorax indicating a pneumothorax. Chest radiograph confirms the pneumothorax when the transillumination is questionable and the infant is stable. A tension pneumothorax is seen readily on radiograph with a large air collection, displacement of the mediastinum away from the air, and collapse of the involved lung. Smaller pneumothoraces are seen as a lucency at the lung periphery or extending above the heart medially. This must be distinguished from a pneumomediastinum, which classically reveals a hyperlucent rim of air lateral to the cardiac borders and thymus and elevates the thymus away from the pericardium, making a "sail sign." Evacuation of a pneumothorax is required if it under tension or if it is compromising the infant's ability to ventilate. Under sterile conditions, a chest tube is placed into the pleural space in the anterior axillary at the fifth intercostal space with a small skin incision. The chest tube is then connected to an underwater seal at suction pressures of 10 to 20 cm H_2O. If the infant is able to adequately ventilate without cardiovascular compromise the infant may be observed and the air collection allowed to resorb. This can be hastened by placing the infant in 100% oxygen, creating a nitrogen gradient between the gas in the pneumothorax and that in the lungs.

Meconium Aspiration Syndrome

Term infants exposed to hypoxic stress in utero may pass a meconium bowel movement before birth, thus contaminating the amniotic fluid. If hypoxia persists, fetal gasping can occur that will draw the meconium-stained fluid into the pharynx and lungs. If further hypoxia has not occurred, the meconium lies predominately in the nose and mouth. When meconium-stained fluid is noted before delivery, the obstetrician suctions the mouth and nose after delivery of the head to prevent the fluid from being drawn into the lungs with the first breaths. Further clearing of the airway and pharynx can be accomplished immediately after birth by intubation and subsequent suctioning with an endotracheal tube. Endotracheal suctioning should be done in the presence of thick meconium or when the infant is depressed and needs resuscitation. Despite these preventive efforts, meconium-stained fluid can enter the lungs, most commonly as a result of in utero fetal gasping, resulting in a chemical pneumonia. The infant initially may appear well, but develops symptoms in the first few hours of life, including tachypnea, cyanosis, grunting, and retractions. A chest radiograph may show coarse, patchy infiltrates and hyperinflation. The severity of the lung disease often does not correlate with the severity of the radiograph. Treatment consists of respiratory support to maintain adequate oxygenation and ventilation. Both the clinical and radiographic picture of meconium aspiration syndrome can be indistinguishable from neonatal pneumonia; therefore, the infant must be evaluated for infection and treated with antibiotics.

Persistent Pulmonary Hypertension of the Newborn

Persistent pulmonary hypertension of the newborn (PPHN) can occur as a primary process or as a complication of other pulmonary processes such as pneumonia, meconium aspiration syndrome, or congenital diaphragmatic hernia. The normal transition at birth from a fetal circulatory pattern to a mature pattern requires a decrease in the pulmonary vascular resistance, with subsequent closure of the ductus arteriosis and foramen ovale. This is facilitated by air entry into the lungs with resultant increase in oxygenation, which acts to decrease pulmonary vascular resistance and constrict the ductus. When adequate oxygenation doesn't occur because of the underlying pulmonary process, the pulmonary vascular resistance remains high, and a right-to-left shunt occurs across the foramen ovale and through the patent ductus arteriosis. This further aggravates hypoxia, resulting in a complicated cycle. Pulmonary vascular pressures remain systemic or suprasystemic. Treatment for PPHN includes placing the infant in 100% oxygen to improve oxygenation. Systemic blood pressure should be maintained in high normal levels (mean arterial pressures of 50 to 70) to minimize the gradient between the right and left sides and thus minimize the shunting. This is accomplished by fluid boluses or pressors, such as dopamine. Hypotension increases the right-to-left shunt and worsens the hypoxia. Another stimulus to relax the pulmonary vascular bed is alkalosis. This can be accomplished metabolically by giving sodium bicarbonate to increase the pH. Alternatively, mechanical hyperventilation to decrease $paCO_2$ and increase the pH will also relax the pulmonary vasculature. Hyperventilation with $paCO_2$ below 20 should be avoided because this will constrict cerebral blood flow in an already compromised infant. Arterial blood sampling or placement of a pulse oximetry probe in a site supplied with preductal blood flow, such as the right radial artery, falsely may give elevated oxygen readings because it has not yet mixed with the poorly oxygenated blood shunted across the duct. Simultaneously measuring from pre- and postductal sites can indicate if shunting is present, with a drop off in oxygenation indicating a significant shunt. Additional therapies for PPHN are currently under investigation. Nitric Oxide is a potent vasodilator, which when inhaled acts selectively on the pulmonary vascular bed. Surfactant also is being evaluated in term infants with a variety of underlying pulmonary disorders. When maximal therapy has been attempted and hypoxia persists, eligibility for extracorporeal membrane oxygenation (ECMO) is assessed.

Apnea

Apnea is defined as a period during which there is cessation of respiration for at least 10 to 15 seconds, which may be associated with cyanosis, pallor, or bradycardia. This must be distinguished from periodic breathing, which occurs in immature infants with pauses in respiration lasting 5 to 10 seconds followed by 10 to 15 seconds of rapid respiration. Periodic breathing is not a pathologic process and resolves with age. Apnea can be a sign of a systemic process or may represent a primary process. Apnea has been described as a symptom in many illnesses, such as sepsis, hypoxia, anemia, seizures, and hypoglycemia, or may be caused by narcotics given to the mother or the baby. In the preterm infant in whom these causes of apnea have been excluded, the episodes may be the result of apnea of prematurity. Most commonly, preterm infants exhibit a mixed apnea that begins with a central respiratory pause followed by airway obstruction. Treatment with methylxanthines, such as theophylline or caffeine, improves apnea by producing a central stimulatory effect and enhancing diaphragmatic contractility. Theophylline is given as a 5 mg/kg loading dose followed by 1 mg/kg every 8 hours. Therapeutic plasma levels are 5 to 10 g/mL. When apnea persists despite adequate drug levels, CPAP will help decrease the episodes of apnea. CPAP appears to splint the upper airway open, minimizing the airway collapse that causes the obstructive component. Apnea of prematurity decreases in frequency with advancing postnatal age.

CARDIOLOGY

During the first week of life, the cardiovascular system undergoes dynamic changes. The pulmonary vascular resistance continues to gradually decrease, and the ductus arteriosis constricts and closes on the third day of life. Often, murmurs heard on the first day of life are caused by these dynamic processes rather than cardiac disorders. In contrast, significant heart disease may be masked by ductal flow and may not become symptomatic until the ductus arteriosis closes. Examples of ductal dependent lesions are hypoplastic left heart syndrome and critical coarctation of the aorta. Other forms of congenital heart disease that result in excessive left-to-right flow, such as a large ventriculoseptal defect or endocardial cushion defect, will not develop signs of congestive heart failure until 1 to 2 weeks of age when the pulmonary vascular resistance has decreased and allows significantly increased pulmonary flow. Murmurs caused by left-to-right shunting may not be heard on initial examination and only become apparent after 2 to 3 days of life. Additional findings in the cardiac examination, such as a hyperactive precordium or discrepancy of pulses between the upper and lower extremities, determine the presence of an underlying cardiac lesion. Cyanotic heart disease with cyanosis that is unresponsive to oxygen presents immediately after birth. Evaluation of possible congenital heart disease should include a hyperoxia test, if cyanotic, four extremity blood pressures, a chest radiograph to assess cardiac size and pulmonary vasculature, an electrocardiogram to evaluate the axis, and an echocardiogram.

Patent Ductus Arteriosis

In preterm infants, the ductus arteriosis can reopen, particularly if there is fluid overload, hypoxia, or acidosis. Clinically, the infant may present with an increasing oxygen requirement, hepatomegaly, tachypnea, and bounding pulses. A wide pulse pressure is noted on blood pressure measurement. This wide pulse pressure may give rise to palmar pulses that are palpable when you gently place your fingertip in the palm of the infant. A more silent presentation may occur with the only manifestation being increased frequency of apneas. The classic machine-like murmur associated with a patent ductus arteriosis in older children is not present. Frequently, a soft systolic murmur is heard along the left sternal boarder and may only be heard intermittently. Conservative therapy with fluid restriction may allow some ducts to close, but the closure often only is transient. Indomethacin promotes duct closure and is most effective in the first 2 weeks of life. Doses of 0.2 mg/kg are given intravenously every 12 hours for three doses. Additional longer courses of 0.1 mg/kg every 12 hours for 5 days improves closure rates without increasing side effects. Indomethacin is contraindicated in acute, severe intraventricular hemorrhage, thrombocytopenia, or when there is evidence of poor renal function, particularly if the creatine is over 1.5 mg/dL. Side effects include decreased urine output with an increase in creatine and risk of bleeding. In term infants, a patent ductus arteriosis is often asymptomatic and can be observed for spontaneous closure. When symptoms persist in term or preterm infants despite medical treatment, surgical ligation is required.

Congestive Heart Failure

Infants with congestive heart failure present with tachypnea and hepatomegaly, caused by an underlying pathologic process. A chest radiograph usually reveals pulmonary edema and cardiomegaly. The time of onset of congestive heart failure provides insight into the possible causes. Congestive heart failure that is evident at birth is the result of high output failure. This may be caused by severe anemia or large arteriovenous shunting from a large arteriovenous malformation in the vein of Galen or in the liver. Presentation of congestive heart failure in the first 2 weeks of life in a preterm infant may signal a patent ductus arteriosis. Congestive heart failure that presents at 2 to 4 weeks of life commonly is caused by congenital heart disease that involves a left-to-right shunt, which has increased shunting as the pulmonary vascular resistence decreases. Preterm infants may develop congestive heart failure in association with chronic lung disease. Treatment includes using diuretics and avoiding fluid overload. Acute treatment with Lasix at doses of 1 mg/kg per dose intravenously or 2 mg/kg per dose po are effective. Chronic treatment with Lasix in preterm infants has been associated with hearing loss, renal calculi, and nephrocalcinosis. Other types of diuretics, such as thiazides and aldactone, can be used as alternatives. All diuretics can cause excessive sodium and potassium excretion and require monitoring of electrolytes.

Hypotension

Defining hypotension in a newborn depends on the size of the infant, with very low birth weight infants having lower normal blood pressure values than term infants. Hypotension is clearly significant when associated with poor pulses or poor perfusion. The causes of hypotension in the newborn are similar to those occuring in older infants and children, including acute blood loss, sepsis, and poor cardiac output. Fluid boluses, such as normal saline or 5% albumin at doses of 10 to 20 mL/kg, can acutely increase the blood pressure, but may cause complications of fluid overload. When repeated fluid doses are required to maintain adequate blood pressure, pressors should be considered. Dopamine, starting at doses of 5 to 10 μg/kg per minute, can be titrated up to achieve stabilization of the blood pressure. Although dobutamine is more effective for increasing cardiac contractility, it can have a paradoxical response of hypotension in newborns.

Hypertension

A diastolic blood pressure greater than 50 mm Hg in preterm and 60 mm Hg in term infants, or a mean pressure of greater than 60 mm Hg in preterm and 70 mm Hg in term infants is beyond the normal range and should be investigated if persistent. Infants with birth weights less than 1500 g account for 25% of the hypertension found in patients admitted to the NICU. This is most commonly a result of prolonged use of umbilical arterial catheters with resultant aortic thrombosis. Prompt removal of the catheter, if still in place, will prevent further propagation of the clot. If an ultrasound does not reveal a clot, further investigation is required. Other causes of hypertension may include renal artery thrombosis, coarctation of the aorta, renal disease, congenital adrenal hyperplasia, hyperthyroidism, narcotic withdrawal, Bronchopulmonary dysplasia, or post-ECMO.

GASTROENTEROLOGY/NUTRITION

Fluid and nutrition play a key role throughout an infant's course in the NICU. In the first days of life, the focus is on providing appropriate fluid intake with attention to glucose and electrolyte balance. Fluid needs vary depending on the infant's gestational age and day of life. Immature infants have increased insensible losses caused by increased water loss through the immature skin. In contrast, newborns of all gestational ages have lower glomerular filtration rates on the first day of life, which slowly increases over the first week of life. All these considerations are weighed when calculating appropriate fluid intake for infants. In immature infants, fluids start at 100 to 120 mL/kg per day and increase to 140 to 160 mL/kg per day by day 3 or 4. In term infants, fluid intake begins at 60 to 80 mL/kg per day, increasing to 120 mL/kg per day by day 3 or 4. Initially only glucose is needed because the infant is born in a relatively fluid-overload state. Sodium and potassium are added after 2 or 3 days or when indicated by following electrolyte values. Electrolytes are not drawn immediately after birth because they are a reflection of maternal values rather than the infant's values. Weight loss is expected for 2 to 3 days in term infants and 5 to 7 days in preterm infants and should not excede 10% of birth weight. Larger amounts of weight loss suggest inadequate fluid intake and dehydration.

Once fluid needs have stabilized, attention must shift to provide nutrition in addition to fluids. Adequate nutrition is essential for infants to allow necessary growth, particularly in the brain. Infants will need 420 to 504 kJ/kg per day for growth. Underlying chronic pulmonary or cardiac disease may result in higher caloric demand and may require 504 to 630 kJ/kg per day for growth. If an infant is unable to be fed enterally, because of either prematurity or an underlying disease process, nutrition should be provided parenterally. Hyperalimentation solutions can provide gradually increasing protein concentrations. Glucose concentrations also can be increased as tolerated. Periphal veins can tolerate up to 12.5% glucose. Centrally placed venous lines can be increased to 20%

glucose to maximize caloric intake. Essential fatty acids must be provided through lipid emulsion. Fats also can be used to increase caloric intake, given in amounts of 2 to 3 g/kg per day. Providing parenteral nutrition can cause complications. Intravenous access with the resultant risk of infection and thrombosis is necessary. Prolonged exposure to hyperalimentation can cause cholestatic liver disease and possible liver failure.

Optimal nutrition is best provided enterally because it allows higher caloric intake with less risk of fluid overload and avoids the need for intravenous lines. In preterm infants and in any term infants who have experienced hypoxia or decreased perfusion, the gastrointestinal tract may not be able to digest fully and absorb the nutrition. When respiratory and cardiac issues have stablized, enteral feeds are slowly introduced. In preterm infants (birth weight less than 1000 g) or older infants who have had significant compromise, the feeds start at 10% of full feeds and are increased over 7 to 10 days. In more mature preterm infants and less compromised term infants, initial feeds can be 20% of full volume and increased over 3 to 5 days. Many choices exist for the type of nutrition to use. Breast milk provides an excellent source of nutrition with the addition of maternal antibodies. When breast milk is not available, a variety of commercial formulas that come as a standard formula or a premature formula can be used. Premature formulas have the higher vitamin, calcium, and caloric content needed by preterm infants. In addition, a larger percentage of the fat is provided as medium chain triglycerides, which are absorbed easily without requiring further breakdown. Standard formulas and breast milk provide 84 kJ/30 mL of formula, whereas preterm formulas have 100.8 kJ/30 mL. When using breast milk in preterm infants, fortifiers can be added that increase the calories and the calcium intake. Preterm infants are iron deficient and fat soluble vitamin deficient as infant stores are accrued in the third trimester. When infants are tolerating full feeds, multivitamin and iron supplements are added.

At gestational ages less than 34 weeks, infants are unable to coordinate suck and swallow, and thus are dependent on gavage feeds. Initial feedings in preterm infants can be started as slow continuous infusions to maximize feeding tolerance. In infants less than 1500 g, feedings are given every 2 hours; in those greater that 1500 g, feeds may be given every 3 hours. Adequate caloric intake is assessed by documented weight gain. Infants receiving full calories should gain 20 to 30 g per day, and head circumference should increase by 1 to 2 cm per week. Inadequate growth indicates the need for additional calories. If additional fluid cannot be tolerated, caloric density of the formula can be increased to provide the additional calories.

Intestinal Obstruction

Infants with an intestinal obstruction may have a prenatal history remarkable for polyhydramnios. Amniotic fluid normally is swallowed by the fetus, but this is impaired in an infant with obstruction. Large amounts of oral secretions in the delivery room may be noted. The infant may present with emesis and poor feeding shortly after birth. Placement of a nasogastric tube decompresses the stomach and also assesses the patency of the esophagus. A radiograph showing the tube curled in the upper thorax would suggest esophageal atresia. The classic radiograph of the "double bubble" consisting of a dilated stomach and a dilated proximal duodenum indicates duodenal atresia. Other forms of obstruction include atresias at other sites in the GI tract, malrotation with volvulus, meconium ileus, and meconium plug syndrome. Meconium ileus, caused by inspissated meconium, is associated with cystic fibrosis. Meconium plug syndrome, also caused by tenacious plugs of meconium, is diagnosed and treated with a gastrograffin enema. The hyperosmolar solution allows loosening and passage of the plugs. Although meconium plug syndrome can be associated with cystic fibrosis, it more commonly is associated with Hirschsprungs disease. All other causes of obstruction require surgical intervention.

Malrotation

When the gastrointestinal tract if formed with inadequate stability of the duodenum, the intestines have increased mobility and can twist around the blood supply. Ischemia and subsequent necrosis of the bowel, called volvulus, can occur if unrecognized. Infants with malrotated intestines can present at any time with volvulus. Onset of emesis, particularly when bilious, should alert one to the possibility of volvulus. Symptoms can appear intermittently or be present shortly after birth. Because of the severity of the outcome, infants with bilious emesis should have an upper GI series to assess the position of the duodenum. Malrotation with volvulus requires prompt surgical intervention to minimize the gut ischemia and to avoid gut necrosis with resultant short bowel.

Necrotizing Enterocolitis

Necrotizing enterocolitis (NEC) is a severe bowel disease that can lead to necrosis, perforation, subsequent short bowel, or death. NEC is a multifactorial disease that results in bacterial invasion of the intestinal mucosa with gas production. This intramucosal air, called pneumatosis, is the classic diagnostic feature of NEC. Pneumatosis can be seen on abdominal radiographs as linear lucencies. More ominous radiographic signs include portal air and pneumoperitoneum indication perforation. Risk factors for NEC include prematurity, previous history of hypoxia or poor gut perfusion, and enteral feeds. Ninety-five percent of all cases of NEC are in infants who have been fed. The greatest risk occurs in infants who have had their feeds advanced by more than 20 mL/kg per day increments. The enteral nutrition provides substrate for bacterial overgrowth.

Clinically, infants may present acutely with grossly bloody stools, abdominal distension and tenderness. More subtle presentations may include apnea and bradycardia, guaiac positive stools, and presence of poor gastric motility manifested by residual gastric contents after feeds. Signs of sepsis also may occur, such as hypotension, poor perfusion, and lethargy. Laboratory findings can include neutropenia, thrombocytopenia, anemia, and metabolic acidosis. Treatment of the infant requires stopping all feeding, assessing for sepsis, and treating with antibiotics, with attention to coverage for GI flora. Additional supportive care is given as required for stabilization. Frequently, infants require intubation because of hypoventilation caused by the abdominal distension. Surgery is indicated only when there is evidence of perforation or necrotic bowel. Persistent acidosis and thrombocytopenia despite improving clinical status may be caused by necrotic bowel. Infants are kept NPO for 7 to 14 days to allow mucosal healing. Long-term complications include malabsorption, failure to thrive, strictures, and short bowel when surgical resections have been required.

HEMATOLOGY

Anemia

Normal hematocrit values in term infants range from 45 to 60% and from 40 to 50% in preterm infants. Infants born with lower levels are anemic commonly caused by acute blood loss, or hemolysis. Acute blood loss can occur because of placenta previa, abruption, cord accidents, or delayed cord damping with the infant elevated from the placenta. Before delivery, the infant can hemorrhage into the placenta and maternal circulation, creating a fetal to maternal hemorrhage. This should be suspected when there is evidence of acute blood loss, but there is no other history of blood loss at delivery. Diagnosis is made by performing a Kleihauer-Betke test on the mother, which quantitates fetal blood on a maternal smear. Treatment for acute blood loss includes fluid resuscitation for symptomatic infants followed by transfusion of packed red blood cells. Asymptomatic infants with less severe anemia can be observed, but may present later with symptomatic anemia. Hemolytic anemia may present at birth, such as with Rh incompatibility, or may develop in the first 24 to 48 hours of life in other forms of blood group incompatibility. Knowing the maternal blood type and antibody screen allows one to anticipate significant hemolytic processes. Mothers with O blood type are at risk for having babies with ABO incompatibility. Additional minor blood group antibodies, such as Lewis or Kell antibodies, are usually detected on the maternal antibody screen. In all mothers with O blood type and those with positive antibody screens, cord blood should be sent to determine the infant's blood type and a direct Coombs test should be performed. Positive direct Coombs test results indicate the presence of antibodies in the infant, which places the infant at risk for hemolysis. When the Coombs test is positive, serial hematocrits must follow to assess for progression of anemia. A high reticulocyte count also suggests a hemolytic process. Treatment depends on the severity of the anemia and the associated increase of bilirubin. Because the infant has not undergone volume loss and may present in high output failure, packed red cell transfusion may aggravate the congestive heart failure.

Polycythemia

Infants exposed to chronic hypoxia in utero may respond by increasing their hematocrit. This occurs most commonly in growth-retarded infants, infants of diabetic mothers, and large for gestational age infants. A hematocrit of greater than 70 in an asymptomatic infant, or a hematocrit of greater than 65 in a symptomatic infant requires intervention. Symptoms include respiratory distress, cyanosis, hypoglycemia, lethargy, poor feeding, or apnea. The symptoms are thought to be caused by sludging of the high-viscosity blood in small vessels. The reason for treatment is because of the risk of blood vessel occlusion and ischemia. Treatment consists of a partial volume, or dulitional exchange transfusion, giving 5% albumin or plasminate while withdrawing an equal volume of blood from the infant to decrease the hematocrit acutely. The volume of exchange is calculated using the estimated blood volume, observed hematocrit, and desired hematocrit.

Neutropenia

Neutropenia is defined by an absolute neutrophil count of less than 1000. The most common cause is bacterial sepsis, in which infants may tend to have neutropenia rather than an elevated white blood cell count. Neutropenia at birth also can be a consequence of severe maternal preeclampsia to eclampsia. Later presentations of neutropenia are commonly the result of a viral infection including cytomegalovirus.

Thrombocytopenia

A platelet count of less than 100,000 denotes thrombocytopenia. Risk of spontaneous hemorrhage becomes of concern when the platelet count is less than 20,000. A theoretical concern exists of increased risk of intraventricular hemorrhage in preterm infants with platelet counts of 20,000 to 50,000. Thrombocytopenia at birth can occur in a variety of conditions. Infections, particularly bacterial sepsis, can cause disseminated intravascular coagulation (DIC) with thrombocytopenia. Autoimmune thrombocytopenia in the mother, such as Idiopathic Thrombocytopenic Purpura (ITP), can have antibody passage across the placenta with resultant thrombocytopenia in the fetus. These infants are at risk of spontaneous intraventricular hemorrhage in utero. The trauma of the birth process also can place the infant at risk for hemorrhage, particularly intracranial hemorrhage. Maternal treatment with IVIG can decrease antibody load before delivery. Cesarean delivery is frequently recommended to minimize trauma to the infant. Isoimmune thrombocytopenia occurs in mothers who are PLA-1 antigen negative and the fetus is PLA-1 antigen positive; the maternal antibodies will cause thrombocytopenia in the fetus with risk of hemorrhage in utero or at delivery. Unlike mothers with ITP who have a low platelet count, mothers who are PLA-1 antigen negative are asymptomatic with normal platelet counts and are not aware of their platelet antibody status before birth.

Infants diagnosed with thrombocytopenia should be evaluated for sepsis. Additionally, urine for cytomegalovirus culture should be sent. Maternal platelet counts are reviewed to look for undiagnosed ITP. If PLA-1 antibodies are suspected, antibody testing on the parents should be performed. Platelet transfusions are done for platelet counts of less than 20,000 or if there are signs of bleeding such as hematuria, guaiac positive stools, or oozing from puncture sites. In both autoimmune and isoimmune thrombocytopenia, random donor platelets may increase the platelet count slightly with a subsequent rapid decrease. If ongoing platelet transfusion is required, maternal platelets provide sustained platelet levels. In most cases of thrombocytopenia, the platelet count gradually returns to normal.

Hyperbilirubinemia

Hyperbilirubinemia is clinically evident as jaundice. In newborns, jaundice is apparent when the bilirubin level is over 5 mg/dL. A transition occurs after birth in bilirubin metabolism. In utero bilirubin is eliminated through the placenta. After birth there is a delay in the onset of hepatic bilirubin metabolism and elimination. This allows a transient or physiologic hyperbilirubinemia over the first several days of life. Jaundice appears on the second or third day of life, peaks at 3 to 5 days in term infants, 5 to 7 days in preterm infants, and subsequently resolves. Levels are not generally above 15 mg/dL total and consists of unconjugated or indirect bilirubin. Physiologic jaundice must be distinguished from pathologic jaundice, which is usually caused by an underlying pathologic process. Pathologic jaundice should be suspected when there is clinical jaundice (a bilirubin level of over 5 mg/dL) in the first 24 hours of life, an increase in bilirubin levels of greater than 5 mg/dL per day, total bilirubin levels of greater than 15 mg/dL, or a direct bilirubin of greater than 2 mg/dL. When pathologic jaundice is suspected, total and direct bilirubin levels are sent. The level is elevated if it is greater than 5 mg/dL in the first 24 hours of life, greater than 10 mg/dL at 24 to 48 hours, or greater than 15 mg/dL at over 48 hours. Additional information is needed to determine the cause and treatment of the hyperbilirubinemia.

Causes for indirect hyperbilirubinemia can be divided into categories of increased production or decreased elimination. Bilirubin is derived from the breakdown of heme. Excess destruction of red blood cells leads to increased bilirubin production. One cause of increased red cell breakdown is hemolysis. Reviewing maternal blood type and antibody screens can determine which infants are at risk for ABO, Rh, or other minor blood group incompatibilities. Further evidence for a hemolytic process can be seen with a low hematocrit, high reticulocyte count, and hemolysis on blood smear. Sending blood type and direct Coombs test on the cord or infant blood further determines the presence of incompatibility. When a hemolytic process is suspected, but there is no predisposing blood group set up, and the Coombs test results are negative, other causes of hemolysis should be considered, such as red cell membrane and enzyme defects. When the hyperbilirubinemia appears to be nonhemolytic, other sources of excess red cell breakdown are investigated. Polycythemia can cause hyperbilirubinemia because of the larger red cell mass. Excessive bruising or large hematomas, particularly large cephalohematomas or intraventricular hemorrhages, can lead to hyperbilirubinemia. Bilirubin is eliminated after hepatic uptake, conjugation, secretion into the biliary tree and, subsequently, into the GI tract where bilirubin is excreted in the stool. Some bilirubin is reabsorbed, which is known as enterohepatic circulation. When oral intake is poor or GI motility is decreased, such as with ileus or obstruction, excessive bilirubin is reabsorbed causing hyperbilirubinemia. Liver disease, which impairs bilirubin uptake or conjugation, also can increase serum bilirubin levels. Another cause of hyperbilirubinemia occurs in breast fed infants. Typically, breast-milk jaundice develops more gradually, peaks at 10 days, and slowly resolves; infants otherwise appear healthy. Stopping breast milk intake for 24 hours with substitution of formula causes a dramatic decrease in serum bilirubin and does not recur after restarting breast milk. Metabolic diseases, such as galactosemia or hypothyroidism, may be associated with hyperbilirubinemia.

High bilirubin levels can result in bilirubin crossing the blood–brain barrier, causing a form of encephalopathy known as kernicterus. This is associated with later development of choreoathetoid cerebral palsy and hearing impairment. The serum bilirubin level at which kernicterus occurs is unclear. Acidosis, hypoxia, hypoalbuminemia, and prematurity are other factors that can cause increased permeability of the blood–brain barrier. Historically, most cases of high bilirubin levels (over 20 mg/dL), with subsequent kernicterus, occurred in hemolytic disease, particularly Rh incompatibility. Preterm infants have been found to have kernicterus on autopsy at much lower levels of bilirubin, e.g., 10 mg/dL in extremely low birth weight infants. With the advent of RhoGAM to prevent sensitization of Rh-negative women, the incidence of kernicterus has decreased significantly. This has led many to believe that bilirubin levels over 20 mg/dL in hyperbilirubinemia from nonhemolytic causes in term infants are not associated with kernicterus.

Initial treatment for indirect hyperbilirubinemia is phototherapy. Bilirubin absorbs ultraviolet light in the blue-green wavelengths, is converted to a more water soluble form, and is excreted in the urine. Adequate hydration must be maintained because phototherapy increases insensible losses. Phototherapy is indicated for hemolytic hyperbilirubinemia with a rapid increase in bilirubin greater than 5 mg/dL per day or at bilirubin levels of 18 to 20 mg/dL in term infants with nonhemolytic disease. In preterm infants, phototherapy should be considered at lower levels, such as 5 to 7 mg/dL at 500 to 1000 g, 7 to 10 mg/dL at 1000 to 1500 g, and 10 to 15 mg/dL at 1500 to 2500 g. In hemolytic disease with rapidly increasing bilirubin levels despite phototherapy, intravenous immunoglobulin decreases the degree of hemolysis. When bilirubin continues to increase despite therapy, and bilirubin levels are nearing those associated with kernicterus, an exchange transfusion is done. This allows removal of both bilirubin and antibodies involved in hemolysis. Exchange transfusions are recommended in term infants at bilirubin levels of over 25 mg/dL in nonhemolytic processes and over 20 mg/dL in hemolytic processes. In preterm infants, exchange transfusions levels are lower because of the increased permeability of the blood–brain barrier. Exchange transfusions should be considered at levels of 12 to 15 mg/dL for 500 to 1000 g infants; 15 to 18 mg/dL at 1000 to 1500 g infants; and at 18 to 20 mg/dL at 1500 to 2500 g infants. The volume of blood exchanged is double the calculated blood volume of the infant. Physicians must be aware of the considerable risk when deciding to perform the exchange transfusion. An arterial line or umbilical venous line is required to perform the procedure. Complications may include hypocalcemia, hypoglycemia, thrombocytopenia, neutropenia, blood pressure instability, and cardiac arrest.

When hyperbilirubinemia has a large direct fraction and direct bilirubin levels greater than 2 mg/dL, a different course of treatment and evaluation must be undertaken. Direct, or conjugated bilirubin, does not cross the blood–brain barrier and thus does not pose a risk of kernicterus. Likewise, phototherapy is not effective in altering conjugated bilirubin into a form that can be excreted and will not decrease the bilirubin level. Phototherapy causes a binding of the direct bilirubin in the skin, resulting in a bronze color. This is a cosmetic problem that does not harm the infant. Direct hyperbilirubinemia can be associated with urinary tract infections; therefore, a urine culture is recommended as part of the evaluation. Liver disease, such as any viral hepatitis (A, B, C, CMV), α-1 antitrypsin, hepatic injury from hypoxia, or chemical hepatitis from prolonged hyperalimentation, can cause a direct hyperbilirubinemia. Obstructions of the biliary tree, such as gallstones or biliary atresia, also can cause a direct hyperbilirubinemia. When presented with an infant with direct hyperbilirubinemia, evaluation should include a urine bacterial culture, a urine CMV culture, liver enzymes, a hepatitis serology, and a liver ultrasound. An absent gallbladder on ultrasound suggests biliary atresia; however, the presence of a gallbladder does not exclude it. A nuclear medicine scan for biliary excretion, such as a HIDA scan, is required to assess the function of the biliary tree. When lack of excretion into the bile duct is found, a liver biopsy is required to confirm or rule out biliary atresia.

RENAL

Infants have lower glomerular filtration rates at birth that gradually increase over the first week of life. Additionally, preterm infants have immature renal function with decreased ability to concentrate. These factors have direct implication for dosing any renally excreted drug. Doses must be adjusted for degree of prematurity and age of the infant. Normal urine output for the first 24 hours in an infant can be as low as 1 mL/kg per hour. Failure to void in the first 24 hours should prompt an investigation of the urinary tract and renal function.

In utero, poor urine output is manifested as decreased amniotic fluid volume. When decreased amniotic fluid volume is prolonged and severe, the fetus is compressed in the uterus and is unable to move freely or undergo fetal breathing movements. Extremities develop contractures, and lack of fetal breathing leads to pulmonary hypoplasia. The faces have a characteristic appearance of a flattened nose and low-set ears. These findings are called the potter syndrome, which usually is lethal because of the pulmonary hypoplasia. Potter syndrome is the end result of any form of renal disease that results in minimal urine output in utero. It also can be seen in prolonged, early, ruptured membranes. Causes of minimal or no urine output in utero include renal agenesis, renal dysplasia, or urinary tract obstructions.

Poor urine output postnatally, in the absence of a history of oligohydramnios, is likely caused by acute tubular necrosis as a result of hypoxia or hypoperfusion of the kidneys. Clinically, the infant will be oliguric with hematuria or occasional anuria and will have increasing urea nitrogen and creatine. Management includes support of oxygenation and perfusion to avoid further injury. Fluid intake must be restricted to compensate for the decreased urinary losses. Close monitoring of electrolytes, particularly potassium, is required. All renally excreted drugs must be followed with serum levels to assure proper dosing. Commonly, after a period of oliguria, recovery may be preceded by polyuria. Again, fluid and electrolyte balances become the focus of management. The majority of infants have gradual recovery of renal function.

INFECTIOUS DISEASE

Newborn infants are susceptible to a variety of infections because of lower levels of activity in their immune systems. Additionally, preterm infants have lower levels of antibodies because the majority of maternal antibodies transfer in the third trimester. Infants can acquire infections prenatally via a hematogenous route through the placenta. Other infections are acquired by ascending through the vaginal canal into the uterine cavity. Maternal history of infections acquired during pregnancy (e.g., herpes, syphilis) can alert one to the risk of infection in the infant. Signs of infection in the mother at the time of birth, such as fever, high white blood cell count or uterine tenderness, places the infant at increased risk of infection. Prolonged rupture of membranes, particularly greater than 24 hours, is associated with increasing risk of infection in the newborn. Additional signs of distress in the infant, such as fetal tachycardia, meconium-stained fluid, or abnormal fetal heart rate patterns, can be associated with infections. After birth, sepsis can present as fulminant septic shock or may have a subtle presentation. Infants may have a fever, but more commonly they are hypothermic or have temperature instability. Clinical features may include lethargy, poor feeding, irritability, tachypnea, apnea, or poor perfusion cyanosis. These features are not specific, and infection frequently must be differentiated from a variety of other illnesses. A blood culture is essential for diagnosing bacterial sepsis, but can be falsely negative in a newborn whose mother was treated with antibiotics more than 4 hours before delivery. A complete blood count can be helpful in distinguishing sepsis from other diseases. Normal white cell counts in newborns range from 5,000 to 30,000. Both leukocytosis and neutropenia can be seen in sepsis, with neutropenia being a more ominous sign. A differential with a left shift or more immature neutrophil forms is associated with sepsis. This shift can be quantitated in an immature to total (I:T) ratio. The ratio is calculated by adding the absolute number of immature forms, such bands and metamyelocytes, and dividing by the total absolute neutrophil count. A ratio greater than 0.2 indicates an increased risk of infection. For example, a differential with 25 polys, 5 bands has an I:T ratio of 5 divided by 30, or 0.17, which is reassuring. A differential of 30 polys, 10 bands has an I:T ratio of 10 divided by 40, or 0.25, which places the infant in a higher risk category for sepsis. Thrombocytopenia can be seen in fulminant sepsis or as part of a congenital viral infection. Urine cultures are not performed in infants less than 3 days of age because urinary tract infections are rare in this age group. After 3 days of age, a urine culture is part of the evaluation for sepsis in infants. Chest radiographs evaluate for pneumonia because specific pulmonary findings are often absent on the physical examination. The criteria for performing lumbar punctures remain controversial. Meningitic signs are frequently absent in infants less than 1 year old. Spinal fluid cultures are positive in tandem with positive blood cultures. Therefore, when a reliable blood culture has been drawn, many will defer the lumbar puncture. But in cases of invalid blood cultures, such as in the case of maternal antibiotic pretreatment, reviewing results of a spinal tap must be done. Spinal fluid in newborns can have up to 20 white blood cells and still be considered normal. Glucose values should be two thirds that of a serum glucose level. Bloody spinal taps are difficult to interpret.

Bacterial Infection

The most common bacterial pathogens in the newborn period are group B β-hemolytic streptococcus, E. Coli, and Listeria. All of these pathogens have two clinical presentations: early onset sepsis and late onset sepsis. Early onset sepsis occurs in the first 3 days of life, usually acquiring the pathogen from the mother perinatally. Early onset sepsis in infants frequently presents with respiratory symptoms, such as tachypnea, grunting, flaring, and retractions with cyanosis, although most infants do not have pneumonia as part of the illness. Additional signs of sepsis, such as pallor, poor perfusion, and lethargy, can develop. Meningitis is uncommon, and early onset disease is seen more frequently in preterm than term infants. Late onset disease presents at 3 to 6 weeks of life. The onset is typically more insidious, with poor feeding and lethargy. Sepsis can be associated with a focus such as cellulitis, arthritis, osteomyelitis, or meningitis.

There is no predisposition for term versus preterm infants. Group B streptococcal disease is by far the most predominant cause of bacterial sepsis. It can be cultured from 30% of all women. Attempts to eradicate the organism from the genital tract are poor because of the reservoir of the organism in the GI tract. Identifying woman colonized by group B streptococcus allows obstetricians to treat the women with penicillin or ampicillin during labor, which has greatly reduced the cases of group B streptococcal sepsis. Likewise, aggressive treatment of women in preterm labor with antibiotics has reduced group B streptococcal sepsis. Treatment for suspected sepsis, both early and late onset, must provide excellent coverage for streptococcus, E.Coli, and Listeria. Concerns regarding the use of nephrotoxic and ototoxic drugs, such as gentamicin, has led some to use the combination of ampicillin and cefotaxime. When this combination has been used exclusively in nurseries, resistant strains of bacteria have emerged. Usually, cephalosporins are reserved for specific indications such as in patients with renal disease or when there is a need for better central nervous system penetration. When an organism is isolated, therapy can be narrowed based on sensitivities.

Preterm infants with prolonged hospitalizations and need for intravenous access in face of immature immune systems can develop nosocomial infections. These infections tend to occur after 3 weeks of life and are frequently caused by staphylococcus epidermis and, occasionally, staphylococcus aureus. Presentation is frequently more subtle, with increased episodes of apnea, feeding intolerance, ileus, and lethargy. Although Vancomycin provides excellent coverage, the emergence of Vancomycin-resistant enterococcus has dictated more judicious use of the drug. Appropriate antibiotic coverage can vary between institutions and should be based on hospital-based organism sensitivity patterns.

Fungal Injection

Fungal infections, particularly with Candida albicans, can be seen at birth or later in the course of an ill infant as a form of a nosocomial infection. Congenital Candida infections occur predominantly in preterm infants. Candida plaques can sometimes be seen on the placenta. There is also an association between Candida infection in infants and cerclage use in their mothers. The infants may have a reddish hue to their skin. In addition to blood cultures, fungus also may be found in the urine. Evaluation should be done to assess for disseminated fungal disease. Fundoscopic examinations may reveal retinal lesions. A renal ultrasound may demonstrate involvement of the renal parenchyma. A white blood cell count may have significant leukocytosis. When the infection is isolated to the urinary tract, with negative blood cultures and abnormal renal ultrasound, a 7- to 10-day course of Amphotericin B is sufficient. If blood cultures are positive or there is evidence of disseminated disease, a 4- to 6-week course of Amphotericin B is required. If blood cultures remain positive on therapy, 5-flucytosine may be added.

Viral Infections

Many viral diseases can cause illness in the newborn period. The most severe is herpes simplex virus. Herpes is transmitted perinatally, and presents at 5 to 10 days of life. In half of the cases of neonatal herpes, there is no history of herpes in the mother. The highest risk of transmission to the infant occurs with primary herpes infection at the time of delivery, which may be asymptomatic, or may present as only postpartum fever. In women with a known history of genital herpes, transmission rates are very low, most likely because of the previous passage of antibodies to the infant. Herpes infection in infants is divided into three categories: cutaneous, disseminated, and central nervous system disease. Cutaneous disease in infants presents with vesicular lesions, which frequently erupt on the presenting parts or can be at the site of a scalp electrode. The infants will otherwise appear well. The vesicles must be differentiated from other skin lesions, such as bullous erythema toxicum. Viral culture of the vesicle can confirm or rule out herpes, but does not supply the information in a timely frame needed for making clinical decisions. Tsank preparations, done by staining material scraped from the base of the vesicle and examining it under the microscope for multinucleated grant cells, are helpful when results are positive. Direct fluorescent antibody (DFA) for herpes can be done promptly and provides good sensitivity and specificity for making clinical decisions. When herpes is suspected, the treatment is acyclovir at a dose of 10 mg/kg per dose every 8 hours. Mortality is very low for cutaneous herpes simplex, but when untreated, can progress to disseminated or central nervous system disease. Disseminated herpes simplex presents similarly to fulminant bacterial sepsis. Only one third of infants have skin lesions at presentation; therefore, the clinical picture is often confused with bacterial sepsis. The onset of symptoms at 5 to 10 days of life is atypical for both early and late onset bacterial sepsis, which should alert one to the possibility of herpes infection. There is often abnormal liver function tests, evidence of DIC, and pneumonia. There may or may not be associated central nervous system infection. Despite supportive care in addition to acyclovir, mortality remains high at 60%. Herpes also can present as an isolated meningoencephalitis. Infants may present with lethargy, poor feeding, or seizures. Spinal fluid reveals high total protein, elevated red blood cell counts, and elevated white blood cell counts with lymphocytosis on differential. Viral cultures may or may not be positive, but PCR will often reveal the virus. Treatment consists of supportive care and acyclovir. Mortality is 15%, but morbidity is significant, with long-term outcomes including cerebral palsy and mental retardation. Even with prolonged courses of acyclovir, recurrences of skin lesions develop. In children with cutaneous disease, increased episodes of recurrences are associated with increased morbidity.

Congenital Infection

Infections occurring in utero can have serious consequences for the developing fetus that frequently result in growth retardation, microcephaly, CNS injury, and other organ system involvement depending on the infection. These are known as TORCH infections, which stands for Toxoplasmosis, Rubella, Cytomegalovirus, and Herpes. Toxoplasmosis is caused by intercellular protozoan Toxoplasma gondii, which is found in cat feces or in tissues of infected animals such as cattle or sheep. Risk factors include exposure to cat feces, or ingestion of undercooked infected meat. Congenital toxoplasmosis occurs as a result of primary maternal infection during pregnancy. Risk of transmission to the fetus is 40%, but varies with gestational age. The risk of transmission increases with increasing gestational age; however, infection acquired earlier in gestation has more severe clinical manifestations than when acquired later in gestation. The classic presentation is the triad of hydrocephalus, chorioretinitis, and intracranial calcifications, although most infants are asymptomatic at birth. Other characteristics may include intrauterine growth retardation, jaundice, or a maculopapular rash. When unrecognized, the disease can progress and present with late-onset seizures, developmental delay, and hearing loss. Diagnosis is based on serologic testing. A positive IgG for toxoplasmosis may only reflect a history of a maternal infection. A positive IgM in the infant confirms the diagnosis. Additional laboratory findings may include thrombocytopenia and abnormal CSF findings of lymphocytic pleocytosis, hypoglycorrhachia, and elevated protein concentrations. Treatment consists of sulfadiazine at 50 mg/kg twice daily and pyrimethamine 1 mg/kg daily for the first year of life. With treatment, 70% of infants have a normal outcome.

Congenital rubella syndrome occurs after a primary maternal infection during pregnancy. As in toxoplasmosis, risk of infection increases with increasing gestational age, but with more severe clinical manifestations occurring with earlier infections. Infants with congenital rubella have intrauterine growth retardation with subsequent failure to thrive. Half of the infants will have "blueberry muffin spots," which are foci of dermal extramedullary hematopoiesis. Microcephaly, deafness, and cataracts are also common findings. Other findings may include hepatosplenomegaly, jaundice, microphthalmia, or chorioretinitis. Hepatitis, pneumonia, myocarditis, or meningoencephalitis also may occur. When maternal rubella occurs during the first 8 weeks of pregnancy, congenital heart disease can develop. The most common lesion is a patent ductus arteriosis, which also can be associated with pulmonary artery or valvular stenosis. Outcome for congenital rubella syndrome is poor, resulting in three quarters of infants with sensorineural deafness, one fourth with severe mental retardation, and the majority of the remaining survivors with learning disorders and behavioral problems. Diagnosis is based on maternal serology, positive IgM for rubella in the infant, and isolation of the rubella virus from the infant, most commonly from the nasopharynx.

Cytomegalovirus in the most common of the intrauterine infections. Congenital infection can occur in both primary and recurrent maternal CMV. With primary infection, there is a 30 to 40% transmission rate, but only a 1% transmission rate with recurrent infection. Maternal seropositivity increases with age. Fifty to 60% of adult women of middle socioeconomic status are seropositive and 90% of women of lower socioeconomic status are seropositive. Day care centers represent a risk to women who are seronegative. Day care workers have an 11% seroconversion rate per year. Mothers with children in day care have a 15% rate of infection, especially when the child is under 18 months old. Symptomatic congenital infection occurs in only 5 to 10% of infected infants and is usually the result of a primary maternal infection early in gestation. Clinically, these infants are small for gestational age and have hepatosplenomegaly, jaundice, petechiae, or microcephaly. In these infants, 25 to 5% are born prematurely. Lab findings may show thrombocytopenia or a hemolytic anemia and periventricular calcification can be seen. Outcome in infants with symptomatic infection include hearing loss, chorioretinitis, mental retardation, or seizures. In asymptomatic infants, 10 to 15% are at risk for sequelae, predominantly hearing loss. Diagnosis is based on viral isolation usually from urine. Although ganciclovir has been used in HIV and immunocompromised patients, its role in congenital infection is not yet clear and is under investigation.

The incidence of congenital syphilis, which had declined in the 1970s, increased in the 1980s. Syphilis is caused by a spirochete, Treponema pallidum, and can be transmitted with either primary or secondary syphilis during pregnancy. Thirty to forty percent of infected infants are stillborn. One third of infected infants are symptomatic at birth. Clinical manifestations include hepatosplenomegaly, hepatitis with direct and indirect hyperbilirubinemia, and bony changes on radiograph. Anemia, thrombocytopenia, and pneumonia can also be seen. Neurosyphilis may be present, but is not usually clinically apparent. Those infants who are asymptomatic are at risk of their disease progressing to neurosyphilis. Untreated syphilis will progress and can involve dental and bony deformities. Of most concern are the neurologic sequelae of deafness, mental retardation, hydrocephalus, cranial nerve palsies, and seizures. Diagnosis is based on serologic testing. A positive VDRL in the mother will be reflected as a positive VDRL in the infant. If there is documentation of treatment in the mother with a subsequent decrease in VDRL titer, congenital syphilis is unlikely. If the mother was inadequately treated, or the infant's VDRL titer is higher than the mother's, the infant is presumed to have congenital syphilis. A lumbar puncture should be performed in all infants being evaluated for syphilis to look for a reactive CSF VDRL or abnormal CSF protein concentration or cell count. Treatment is with penicillin G, 50,000 U/kg intravenously every 12 hours for 10 to 14 days. Close follow-up of infants is imperative with serial VDRL tests done at 1, 3, 6, and 12 months old. Titers should decline and become nonreactive. If neurosyphilis was present on CSF examination at birth, repeat CSF evaluations should be done at 6-month intervals.

2

Pediatric Intensive Care

Diane C. Lipscomb, Mark A. Helfaer

This chapter reviews a broad range of pathologic conditions that present to a pediatric ICU. Age-related physiologic and metabolic processes are particular to the pediatric ICU. This difference is important in directing appropriate care of the infant or child. More specific and focused therapeutic options regarding approach of the pediatric cardiac patient are presented in another chapter. This introduction explores further the specifics to care of the pediatric patient in an ICU.

HISTORY

All patients requiring an ICU admission need complete histories and physicals. Admissions are distributed into two categories, surgical and medical. In a postoperative patient, the surgical procedure and intraoperative course are necessary information. Other medical problems and any pertinent past history also help in patient management. Children sustaining life-threatening trauma are admitted to the PICU on surgical services. The mechanisms of injury, primary and secondary injuries, and relevant history are vital to the care of the trauma patient.

The *second* group of patients admitted to the PICU are medical patients. Children require critical care monitoring for a variety of illnesses from life-threatening respiratory and infectious illnesses to complications of underlying medical conditions (i.e., cancer, liver failure, etc.). Children presenting with a new condition require a thorough history inquiring into an etiology.

The past medical and surgical histories are very important to all pediatric admissions to the ICU. Understanding the complete illness affords more effective and compassionate care to the child. As always, medications, allergies, and any significant family history (important in metabolic or congenital conditions) are included in the initial history. An accurate list of medications, in milligram or gram doses, helps vastly in the PICU admission process.

Pulmonary

Children may be admitted to the ICU for primary pulmonary disease or respiratory disease secondary to other illnesses. Asthma, pneumonia, ARDS, and croup are common primary issues that may require ICU monitoring. Children also are admitted for respiratory failure following status epilepticus or sepsis and may need respiratory support following an extensive surgical procedure or massive trauma. Daily assessment includes the primary condition, its impact on respiratory management, and therapies to institute or diminish.

In an extubated patient, the stability of the airway is a basic initial assessment. Upper airway obstruction should be evaluated for the etiology (i.e., stridor) and treated with pharmacologic or mechanical maneuvers (i.e., racemic epinephrine or steroids versus intubation). A patient with an unstable airway is an emergency and should be treated aggressively.

After assessing airway issues, breathing or the lower airway is addressed. Patients require different modes of respiratory support depending on the degree of respiratory failure as a result of lower tract disease or neurologic depression. In the nonintubated patient, oxygen is initially applied for hypoxemia. Oxygen is delivered by a cannula, face mask, or nonrebreather mask. A patient receiving 100% oxygen by a well-fitting nonrebreather mask with declining saturations needs evaluation for more invasive respiratory support.

If more support is required, continuous pressure may be delivered by three modes. The first two modes, applied externally, are continuous positive airway pressure (CPAP) with an inspired oxygen percentage (up to 100%) and bilevel positive airway pressure (BiPAP) with inspiratory and expiratory pressure settings. BiPAP usually supplies inspired oxygen at 2 to 3 L/min, but up to 100% FiO_2 may be given. In the pediatric patient, these modes often require some sedation that may adversely affect the respiratory drive.

Finally, a patient may require endotracheal intubation to deliver effectively pressure and oxygen to the lungs. Intubation is indicated when respiratory failure proceeds to severe hypercarbia and/or hypoxemia refractory to noninvasive modes. Higher CO_2 levels may be tolerated in patients as long as respiratory effort is sufficient to allow adequate oxygenation and cardiac output.

Currently, many different ventilators are in use that offer conventional mechanical ventilation in volume or pressure modes, oscillatory ventilation with high mean airway pressures and small tidal volumes, and jet ventilation using lower mean airway pressures. Ventilatory mode decisions are directed by a patient's disease process. Lung compliance reflects the distensibility of the lungs. Normal lungs receive a tidal volume breath with low-peak lung pressures. As a disease process evolves, lungs become less distendible with less volume entering the lungs at higher peak pressures. Volume ventilation delivers a specific volume of breath to a patient. Approximately 10 to 15 mL/kg accounts for dead space ventilation of the ventilator circuit. A peak pressure is measured by the ventilator which depends on a patient's compliance. Alarms are set for high-peak pressures signaling a decrease of the patient's compliance. To limit peak pressures in poorly compliant lungs, pressure ventilation may be instituted. A peak inspiratory pressure (PIP) is set and, depending on flow and compliance, a volume breath is delivered to the patient.

The oxygenation index incorporates fraction of delivered oxygen, mean airway pressure (MAP), and P_AO_2 (Oxygenation index = $FiO_2 \times MAP / P_AO_2$). Higher indexes are found in patients requiring high inflating pressures and inspired oxygen with only marginal arterial oxygen levels. To manage these patients, high frequency oscillatory ventilation may be instituted. The patient receives small breaths at 6 to 8 cycles per second while a high continuous mean airway pressure is maintained. This mode of ventilation is effective in patients with refractory hypoxia because it diminishes the shear forces of pressure limited ventilation that are seen with increasingly higher peak inspiratory pressures. Jet ventilation is similar to oscillatory ventilation but uses lower mean airway pressures. In these modes of ventilation, permissive hypercapnia may also be practiced. In severe lung disease, attempts to normalize CO_2 are detrimental to lungs, because increasing support results in more toxicity to the diseased lungs. By accepting higher CO_2 and lower pH values, secondary trauma to lungs may decrease without increasing morbidity.

In rare cases, these modes of ventilation are unsuccessful in maintaining sufficient oxygenation and ventilation. Extracorporeal membrane oxygenation (ECMO) bypasses the lungs and heart providing the patient with adequate pulmonary function and cardiac output. The patient's disease process may then resolve without the secondary insult from high levels of ventilatory support. ECMO currently is used most frequently in the neonatal population for persistent pulmonary hypertension or meconium aspiration. In cases of severe hypercarbia, a variation of ECMO also is used for CO_2 removal. The inhalational agent nitric oxide currently is under investigation and is being used as a selective pulmonary vasodilator for severe cases of pulmonary hypertension. Nitric oxide may be useful in the neonatal population in decreasing the morbidity seen with the use of ECMO.

The preceding modes of ventilation and pulmonary support have improved mortality and morbidity in the pediatric population with meconium aspiration, pulmonary hypertension, and ARDS. Attempts at normoventilation also have been replaced with permissive hypercapnia. Tolerance of CO_2 levels in the 60s with pH values > 7.25 have permitted the clinician to decrease the toxicity of high ventilatory settings thus improving outcomes.

Various monitors are used in the ICU to follow the respiratory status of patients. Pulse oximetry and co-oximetry measure oxygen saturation in the blood. The mechanism of pulse oximetry gives a "functional" saturation while the mechanism of co-oximetry gives a "fractional" saturation, which is important when met- or carboxyhemoglobin may be present. Pulse oximetry only will read the percentage of saturation of functioning hemoglobin without measuring any dyshemoglobins. Co-oximetry accounts for all hemoglobin types and measures oxygen delivered by all hemoglobin types. Thus, in methemoglobinemia, a pulse oximetry reading of 90% may be actually 70% when the fractional saturation is measured by co-oximetry.

Carbon dioxide levels may also be measured via external monitors. Capnography monitors the end-tidal or end-expiratory fraction of carbon dioxide in mechanically ventilated patients. This monitor is complicated by severe ventilation perfusion mismatches in patients giving erroneous readings or by airway obstruction. In infants, a percutaneous monitor can measure CO_2, but is limited because of the mechanism of heating the skin for accurate readings and thus the monitor needs frequent and careful following. Although, these systems can be excellent noninvasive tools for monitoring, both oxygen and carbon dioxide monitors should be correlated periodically with the gold standard—arterial blood gases. These may be checked peripherally with a digital arterial blood gas or by an arterial line in a peripheral artery (i.e., radial, posterial tibialis, etc.). Chest x-rays are followed as clinically indicated and at least daily in the intubated or critically ill patient.

Cardiac

Cardiac disease in the PICU is vastly different from that of adults. A large majority of heart disease is congenitally acquired lesions that require surgical correction early in life. An extensive discussion of issues regarding these patients is presented in another chapter. Here, a review of cardiac issues in other medical patients is addressed.

Children admitted to the unit with multisystem organ failure can have cardiac dysfunction. Arrhythmias and hypotension are manifestations of myocardial dysfunction. All children are monitored with electrocardiography and frequent or continuous blood pressure measurement. Ischemic changes on a rhythm strip, hypotension with decreased perfusion, or arrhythmias are signs of a poorly performing myocardium in a scenario often with increased requirements.

Arrhythmias are treated according to ACLS protocol. After control of the arrhythmia, an increase of myocardial perfusion and correction of any electrolyte abnormalities is crucial to improve myocardial performance. Hypotension should be treated according to the etiology. In septic conditions, profound hypotension is secondary to a significantly decreased systemic vascular resistance (SVR). Volume replacement and addition of agents to increase SVR are appropriate therapy to increase blood pressure. Norepinephrine and phenylephrine pharmacologically improve vascular tone thus increasing SVR. Often, primary myocardial depression as a result of inflammatory mediators will require inotropic agents, such as dobutamine and epinephrine. In children, dopamine is an excellent agent to improve blood flow to the kidneys and mesenteric organs during hypotension.

Determining the proper inotropic agent can be difficult at times. All the preceding agents can increase the work and energy requirements of the heart; however, careful interpretation of all data is important. In the critically ill patient, continuous cardiac and blood pressure monitoring and careful attention to calcium, magnesium, and phosphorus are vital. Toe temperature compared with central temperatures measure cardiac output and SVR. A significantly decreased temperature represents an increased SVR or decreased cardiac output. A vasodilated vascular bed clinically seen with red flushed skin and increased toe temperatures indicates a decreased SVR. In conjunction with other clinical parameters, these two situations may reflect cold and warm septic shock respectively.

More invasive lines allow the measurement of various parameters that reflect cardiac output and its adequacy. The equation for oxygen delivery reflects the amount of delivered oxygen and the cardiac output. A central venous line allows measurement of venous blood gases and saturations. Normal venous saturations are 65 to 75%. Decreased venous saturation reflects either an increased need with increased extraction or inadequate delivery to the end organs. As per the oxygen delivery equation, decreased cardiac output or decreased oxygenation can be the etiology. Increased venous saturations conversely may reflect over delivery with decreased extraction or dead tissue and no extraction. Cardiac output also can be measured directly using the thermodilution technique, a Swan-Ganz catheter placed into the pulmonary artery that determines cardiac output, SVR, pulmonary vascular resistance, and oxygen extraction. This information helps determine appropriate inotropic or chronotropic support.

Neurologic

Patients admitted to the ICU may have a primary disease of the central nervous system (CNS) (i.e., closed head injury, brain tumor, or seizures) or secondary disease of the central nervous system as a result of a medical illness (coma because of liver disease or inborn errors of metabolism). Management encompasses basic respiratory and cardiac management along with the treatment of CNS disease. The focus of neurologic intensive care is to preserve cerebral blood flow.

A patient's neurologic status is evaluated with a complete neurologic examination and a Glasgow Coma Scale (GCS). A neurologic examination should be as complete as possible. In the comatose patient, sensory examinations are limited as well as the cognitive abilities assessment. Reflexes and strength can be evaluated. Cranial nerve and brain stem examinations are also obtainable and are important in evaluating the comatose closed head injured patient. The GCS determines the degree of coma in patients. Three categories (verbal, motor, and eye) comprise the scale. The maximum score for motor is 6, for verbal is 5, and for eye is 4. An alert, oriented patient will have a score of 15. A brain dead patient will have a score of 3. In pediatrics, the GCS is age modified to adjust for developmental stages. Infants will have a 5 for the verbal score if babbling or crying to the appropriate stimuli. Motor scores may be difficult to determine. Infants and children often become frightened and will have an altered motor response in a trauma situation. The overall assessment is important.

Activity	Adult Response	Score	Infant Response
Eye opening	Spontaneous	4	Spontaneous
	To verbal stimuli	3	To speech
	To pain	2	To pain
	None	1	None
Verbal	Oriented	5	Coos and babbles
	Confused	4	Irritable cries
	Inappropriate words	3	Cries to pain
	Nonspecific sounds	2	Moans to pain
	None	1	None

Motor movements	Follows commands	6	Normal spontaneous
	Localizes pain	5	Withdraws to touch
	Withdraws to pain	4	Withdraws to pain
	Flexion to pain	3	Abnormal flexion
	Extension to pain	2	Abnormal extension
	None	1	None

Patients admitted to the neurosurgical service often have one of the following three problems:

1. Brain tumors requiring resection
2. Intraventricular catheters being placed for increased cerebrospinal fluid (CSF) and pressure
3. Evacuation of extravascular blood whether epi- or subdural

After surgery, these patients are followed postoperatively to evaluate any change in hemodynamic or neurologic status which would require prompt evaluation (CT scan) and/or surgical intervention (subdural or clot removal).

Patients presenting combative, obtunded, or comatose have an expansive differential diagnosis. In the pediatric population, closed head injury, infectious encephalopathies, inborn errors of metabolism, liver disease, drug ingestion, and neurologic disease may all cause a comatose state requiring ICU monitoring. History and physical examination help to differentiate many of these conditions, but the new onset comatose state with minimal history deserves the appropriate metabolic and neurologic workup. The management often is directed by the inciting problem. In patients with medical illness inducing the coma state, management of the primary condition is crucial.

In many patients admitted to the ICU, coma with increased intracranial pressure (ICP) is managed aggressively. Increased ICP results from tissue and cellular edema that can occur in uncontrolled metabolic conditions (i.e., hyperammonemia as a result of liver disease or inborn errors of metabolism and diabetes mellitus) or from trauma with shear injuries or diffuse intraparenchymal bleeding. To manage ICP, placement of an intracranial catheter can be helpful. These catheters may be placed anywhere from an intraventricular to an epidural position, however, the decision for placement is not always straightforward. In many metabolic disorders, ICP monitors do not change outcome and are not used. In head trauma, the benefits are more defined. Patients with a closed head injury without bleeding diathesis and GCS < 8 are candidates for a ICP catheter. Neurosurgeons in the PICU place the catheter.

The goal of ICP management is maintenance of cerebral blood flow. In metabolic disorders, this is best achieved by controlling the underlying condition and maintaining adequate oxygenation and blood pressure. In closed head injuries, therapy is varied but has certain goals. First, an adequate cardiac output for oxygen delivery and maintenance of cerebral perfusion pressure is vital. Patients should be adequately fluid resuscitated. A second management technique increases osmolarity while decreasing body free water by administration of diuretics in the form of mannitol or furosemide. Osmolar therapy with hypertonic saline solutions may also be used. Normal saline (0.9%) and mannitol classically has been used to increase serum sodium and osmolarity. Currently, 1 to 3% saline more aggressively increases serum sodium without vigorous diuresis. With maintenance infusion rates, sodium levels are increased to 150 to 155 and osmolarity to 280 to 310. Ventilatory management is also important in ICP management. Normocapnia should be used at all times. Hyperventilation and hypocapnia are useful for acute spikes in ICP. Chronic use of hyperventilation eventually resets the brain's autoregulatory curve, and the beneficial effect disappears.

Attention to temperature, glucose, sedation, and seizures is also important in managing the patient with increased ICP. Hyperthermia and hyperglycemia have been associated with worsened outcome in head injured patients. The aggressive treatment of increased temperature is vital, and refractory ICP is managed with hypothermia. Glucose levels should be normalized. Insulin should be administered for glucose levels > 200. Seizures need aggressive management with benzodiazepines or phenytoin. In patients with focal bleeding, prophylactic management of seizures often is instituted. Finally, in a patient with severe ICP, a craniotomy to relieve pressure can be considered in the appropriate clinical scenario

Status epilepticus requiring aggressive drug medication often results in a comatose patient. Complicated febrile seizures or breakthrough seizures in a preexisting disorder are two causes of status epilepticus. During status, respiratory effort is ineffective thus requiring supplemental oxygen or airway protection. The benzodiazepines (diazepam or lorazepam) or barbiturates (phenobarbital) administered to stop seizure activity can further depress respiratory drive also requiring airway protection. Subclinical status epilepticus presents as a nonresponsive or comatose patient with history of a seizure disorder who by electroencephalogram (EEG) has continuous seizure activity.

Infections and ingestions also affect a patient's mental status. Meningitis and encephalitis will alter level of consciousness and may progress to cerebral edema and brain death. The prompt diagnosis and treatment are key to decreasing morbidity and mortality. Accidental ingestions in toddlers and suicide attempts in adolescents often involve ingestion of a variety of prescription and/or illegal drugs that effect the neurologic system. Effects can range from sedation to seizures with cardiovascular collapse. Detoxification appropriate to the ingestion should be instituted immediately with symptomatic treatment thereafter.

In addition to the physical examination, various diagnostic tests and monitoring devices are helpful with management. A CT or MRI scan yield information regarding brain tumors, infiltrative processes, bleeding whether intra- or extraparenchymal, and shear injuries. A CT scan cannot determine increased ICP. To accurately monitor pressure intracranially, an intracranial catheter should be placed. EEGs allow monitoring of the brain's electrical activity. Continuous monitoring aids in treatment of subclinical seizures. Finally, evaluation of CSF is important in infectious and neurologic disorders. Exclusion of increased ICP by CT or fundoscopic examination should be done first.

Many metabolic and autonomic derangements may be seen following brain injury. Of these, one of the most difficult to manage and diagnose is the water and salt abnormalities. Least frequently, brain injury may cause the syndrome of inappropriate antidiuretic hormone release (SIADH). More commonly, diabetes insipidus (DI) or cerebral salt wasting (CSW) are seen. SIADH is manifested by decreased urine output with falling serum sodium levels. DI and CSW are manifested by large volumes of urine output but with elevated or decreased serum sodium levels respectively. To differentiate these three syndromes, the following chart is helpful.

Syndrome	Urine-Specific Gravity	Urine Output (mL/kg/hr)	Serum Sodium (mg/dL)
SIADH	> 1.025	< 0.5	120–130
DI	< 1.001	> 2–4	145–155
CSW	< 1.005	> 2– 4	120–130

Urine and serum osmolarities also may be useful in following the course of these syndromes. Patients with SIADH should have careful fluid restriction and attempts to correct sodium levels to the 140 range because of the associated cellular swelling in hyposmolar states. Patients with DI initially require fluid replacement followed by vasopressin replacement therapy. CSW patients require aggressive water and salt replacement. These patients often require 3% saline for 2 to 3 days. In all of these conditions, time resolves the abnormalities and only in the occasional patient with DI will long-term therapy be needed.

Gastrointestinal

The gastrointestinal (GI) system usually is secondarily affected by other illnesses that bring children to the ICU. Only children with liver disease and surgically repaired intestinal obstructions are seen primarily in the ICU. In critical illness, stress responses, poor systemic perfusion, and sedative use adversely affect the GI system with increased gastric acid production and poor GI motility. The GI tract also serves as an important barrier against bacteria, but in the systemically ill patient the GI tract becomes a potential site for bacterial translocation resulting in septicemia.

Children may be admitted to the PICU following repair of bowel obstruction. Obstructions such as intussusception, volvulus, or malrotation may not be immediately evident in a child. Symptoms develop over hours and are difficult to interpret in a nonverbal infant or a babbling toddler. Thus more extensive bowel necrosis and severe dehydration may be present and, children in shock require intensive care monitoring postoperatively.

Liver disease occurs in childhood with obstructive disorders (i.e., biliary atresia) or as a result of hepatitis of viral or metabolic etiology. End-stage disease needs ICU care because of a variety of problems. Liver failure causes decreased production of clotting factors and bleeding may occur. Also, the presence of varicosities in the portal system predisposes these patients for GI bleeding. Ascites compromises respiratory status and may need periodic removal. Hyperammonemic crises require dialysis to remove the toxins that the liver is unsuccessfully removing to prevent irreversible neurologic injury. Renal failure may also be seen in the end-stage liver patient further compromising liver function and requiring dialysis. The ultimate goal for an end-stage liver patient is a transplant. The postoperative management occurs in the PICU.

More commonly in the PICU, GI issues require vigilant maintenance to avoid other problems in critically ill patients. Cushing's and Curling's ulcers are described in the neurosurgical and burn patient population in critical care settings. However, within the ICU, any patient is at risk for increased acid production and ulcer formation with GI bleeding. If possible, gastric pH should be monitored routinely. H_2 blockers (ranitidine or famotidine) should be administered to control acidity in the 5 to 7 pH range. More frequent administration is required than that seen in the outpatient setting (i.e., every 4 to 6 hours). Continuous infusion is also required. Addition of acid neutralizers is helpful in patients tolerating gastric medicines. The neutralization of stomach acid, however, allows the overgrowth of bacteria. Nosocomially-acquired tracheitis or pneumonias may occur secondary to aspiration.

Because of anxiety and painful procedures in the PICU, anxiolytics and narcotics are used frequently. One significant side effect of these medicines is upon GI motility. The decreased transit time in the GI tract also is complicated by the severity of a patient's illness. Maintenance of GI motility is important, however. The addition of gastric motility agents will promote forward contractions. Stool softeners or stimulant agents allow regular bowel movements. The institution of enteral feeds, even at a minimal rate, also helps maintain GI motility. Enterally feeding patients may also help in preventing infection in the ICU. In an unused GI tract, atrophy of the villa occurs allowing translocation of bacteria and fungus into the bloodstream of a patient. Maintenance of this border may afford some protection to critically ill patients.

Renal

Renal dysfunction in the ICU is often secondary to other concurrent medical or surgical issues. Chronic renal failure as a result of primary renal disease rarely requires ICU monitoring except in the post transplant patient. Acute renal failure requiring dialysis can be associated with hemolytic uremic syndrome or newly diagnosed leukemias in tumor lysis syndrome, but most renal failure and dysfunction in the ICU is secondary to overwhelming systemic illness with multisystem organ dysfunction.

Classically, renal failure is classified into three categories: prerenal, renal, and postrenal. Rarely in the ICU will a distal kidney obstruction cause renal failure. More commonly, prerenal or renal causes of failure are present. First, hypotensive and hypovolemic patients will release antidiuretic hormone, atrial natriuretic factor and other mediators that decrease urine output in an effort to maintain intravascular volume. A patient with a deplete intravascular volume as a result of dehydration will have increased antidiuretic hormone release that diminishes urine volume. Repletion of volume will restore urine output correcting *pre*renal failure. However, if prolonged severe hypotension does not resolve, a patient is at risk for acute tubular necrosis (ATN). End-organ ischemia results from insufficient cardiac output and oxygen delivery to the kidneys resulting in sludging within the tubules, development of ATN, and renal failure. Multisystem organ dysfunction commonly results in ATN and the *renal* failure seen in the PICU. Myoglobinuria also causes renal failure in the PICU patient population. Increased myoglobin release is seen after crush or electrocution injuries, prolonged seizures, and in metabolic disorders. The deposition of myoglobin in tubules also causes ATN.

Renal failure may be polyuric, oliguric or anuric. In the polyuric patient, excessive urine output should be replaced. Urine output beyond appropriate hourly and insensible losses can worsen hypovolemia. Decreased urine output may need restriction of fluids as able with close monitoring of respiratory status for pulmonary edema. Hypotension, however, may preclude significant fluid restriction in the critically ill patient.

Life-threatening metabolic derangements may occur during renal failure. Creatinine clearance $< 25\%$ may be associated with the loss of the kidney's ability to effectively excrete potassium and maintain calcium and phosphorous. Restriction of potassium, and monitoring the levels and ratio of calcium and phosphorous with appropriate adjustments are necessary. Uric acid also increases during renal failure. Deposition of uric acid crystals in renal tubules occurs at levels above 15 mg/dL aggravating renal failure, and addition of allopurinol is indicated. If myoglobinuria is present, the urine should be alkalinized to a pH of >7 to increase myoglobin excretion.

Attempts to augment urine output help to maintain urine flow. Conversion of oliguric or anuric renal failure to polyuric may be associated with better renal recovery. Furosemide or mannitol are helpful in sustaining urinary flow. In some cases, a continuous infusion of furosemide is successful. If urinary function can't be managed with diuretics and fluid therapy, dialysis may be instituted. Peritoneal dialysis may be done but requires a surgical procedure and a period of wound healing.

More commonly, intravascular catheters are placed that allow continuous dialysis of the blood with or without ultrafiltration. Hemodialysis may be performed via a continuous veno-venous circuit or an arteriovenous circuit (CVVH, CVVHD or CAVH, CAVHD respectively). These circuits allow withdrawal of blood into an artificial kidney for dialysis and possible ultrafiltration and then return to the body. Heparinization of the patient is needed to prevent thrombosis of the artificial circuit. These modes of dialysis allow hourly adjustment of fluid status and adjustment of metabolic parameters.

Infectious Diseases

As mentioned in previous sections, a variety of infectious illnesses may require intensive care monitoring. Any system in the body may be involved in an infectious process that progresses to sepsis with multiorgan involvement. Pneumonia may progress to respiratory failure. Meningitis or encephalitis can impair cerebral functioning. Kidney infections may progress to urosepsis. Children with other medical illness, especially cancer and immunodeficiencies, are at risk for overwhelming infections during immunosuppressed periods. The management of these and other infections is determined by the most likely bacterial or viral agents. Antibiotic or antiviral therapy is directed accordingly, and supportive care is given according to the systemic response to the illness.

The pediatric ICU has a few infectious diseases that are particular to children and deserve mention. In late fall and winter, respiratory synctival virus (RSV) causes a bronchiolitis in infants and children. It is an aggressive virus that can lead to severe respiratory failure. Children with underlying medical illness (i.e., bronchopulmonary dysplasia, congenital heart disease) are particularly susceptible to this viral disease. Treatment is controversial with unclear efficacy demonstrated with ribavirin. This virus is very contagious and strict regard to appropriate isolation techniques should be followed. With the advent of IVIG for RSV, chronic PICU patients may be candidates to receive this medication to decrease the risk of acquiring.

Bordetella pertussis is a bacterium that causes whooping cough in infants and children. Infants afflicted with pertussis will have severe paroxysms of coughing that are often associated with apnea. ICU monitoring is warranted during the most severe paroxysms. Erythromycin is used for treatment of the patient and any symptomatic family member or exposed individuals. Again, strict isolation is needed until the infective period is over.

For a variety of reasons, patients in the ICU are at risk for nosocomial infections. The presence of invasive lines for inotrope infusion, arterial blood pressure monitors, and endotracheal intubation place a severely stressed body at infectious risk. Bacterial invasion of any of these foreign objects invades directly into the blood stream or the lungs. Antibiotics are often necessary for treatment, but any antibiotic usage allows a generation of resistant bacteria. Many ICUs are plagued by panresistant enterococci and staphylococci. The use of antibiotics also predisposes a patient for fungal overgrowth and infection. If acquired, many fungal infections are associated with a high mortality. Being critically ill also causes a relative decrease in the body's defense mechanisms. To decrease risk of acquired infections, appropriate line care, good hand washing, and attention to nutrition is valuable.

Fluid, Electrolytes, and Nutrition

Fluid administration in the pediatric patient depends on the size of the patient. Infusion rates are determined by the patient's weight or

m^2. A simple formula to calculate maintenance fluid is based on weight in kg. For the first 10 kg, 4 mL/kg per hour is administered. For the second 10 kg, an additional 2 mL/kg per hour is given. Above 20 kg, 1 mL/kg per hour is further administered. The composition of fluids is determined by the age and clinical status of the patient. Age and body fluid composition determine sodium requirements. In the critically ill patient, hyposmolar fluids are inappropriate replacement. Normal saline of or lactated Ringer's should be used for replacement of fluid and for resuscitation. Colloids, such as albumin, also may be used to resuscitate, especially if the patient is hypoalbuminemic. Often, blood products are necessary. Judicious administration of blood products should be done, giving patients the most appropriate replacement while decreasing exposure to multiple donors.

After a patient has had sufficient volume replacement, maintenance fluids are given containing appropriate concentrations of electrolytes. Also, a source of dextrose should be given in these fluids to provide a substrate for metabolism. During the acute phase of the illness, patients may require greater than the hourly maintenance infusion in addition to bolus therapy.

When clinically possible, nutrition should be instituted enterally or parenterally. The benefits of enteral nutrition have been discussed previously. Even a continuous low flow rate, if tolerated, will afford some stimulation to the villous border. If unable to achieve adequate enteral nutrition, parenteral nutrition should be started. Carbohydrates, fat, and protein are begun and advanced per the patient's tolerance. Goal calories vary with each patient and their disease process. A pediatric nutritionist is very helpful in monitoring the tolerance and directing the advancement of parenteral nutrition.

Pain and Sedation

The definition of an ICU is a hospital unit that treats and monitors critically ill patients. As per the preceding discussions, a patient can experience anxiety from the severe illness and need procedures for appropriate monitoring. A patient deserves appropriate sedation and analgesia during this time. For children, the ICU can be very terrifying. The lack of control a child feels and a parent's frustration over their child's illness are very real and important issues in the PICU. To not aggravate their current condition, many children in the PICU require aggressive sedation. Appropriate use of anxiolytics and analgesics are an absolute.

The administration of medication is directed by the clinical scenario. Longer acting benzodiazepines, such as diazepam or lorazepam, help with anxiety and have a long half life. A small dose on a scheduled basis helps maintain a level of sedation. Narcotics often are used to treat pain in the ICU. Many patients have medical or surgical conditions requiring minimal agitation. Often high doses of narcotics and benzodiazepines are administered for anesthesia because of tolerance phenomena. As the illness improves, many patients will need a gradual reduction of medications to prevent withdrawal.

Although intravenous anesthesia is fairly common in the PICU, inhalation agents are rarely seen. The rare indication for anesthesia in the PICU is status asthmaticus. In this clinical scenario, the inhalational agents are used as a potent bronchodilator in the worst cases of bronchospasm. Local anesthesia is used for procedures such as line placement, chest tube placement, or minor surgical procedures such as suturing or reduction of broken limbs.

Neuromuscular blockers infrequently are used in the PICU on a regular schedule. Only the rare postoperative congenital heart disease repair or children with severe lung disease require around the clock paralysis. Long-term use of neuromuscular blockades are associated with a prolonged muscular weakness that persists after discharge from the ICU. The neurologic examination of the patient is also eliminated in the paralyzed patient and, in many critically ill children, routine neurologic checks are vital in assessing cortical function. Because of these disadvantages, neuromuscular blockade is limited in the PICU. Aggressive use of sedation is preferred.

Hematology and Oncology

Many patients admitted to the ICU will have underlying hematologic or oncologic disorders. Patients with sickle cell disease may have sickle cell crises that threaten life. Acute chest syndrome is an example. Children with cancer have periodic neutropenia that predisposes them to overwhelming and life-threatening infections requiring ICU supportive services. Children status post bone marrow transplants also are at risk for sepsis as well as other post bone marrow complications such as mucocytis, veno-occlusive disease, or graft versus host that may require ICU supportive services.

Patients with sickle cell disease often have bone crises that are managed with fluids and pain management. Some manifestations of crisis however require more aggressive intervention to prevent loss of tissue or life. Priapism and extensive surgical procedures are indications for double volume exchange therapy. Acute chest syndrome happens when sickle cells occlude the lungs, which leads to infiltrates, progressive hypoxemia, and potential respiratory failure. The diagnosis is hypoxia in room air, abnormal CXR, and respiratory distress. The patient's blood volume is withdrawn and sickle-free blood is replaced twice. The formula for exchange is as follows:

$$\text{Vol of packed RBC} = \frac{2 \times \text{patient's Hct} \times \text{patient's estimated blood volume}}{\text{Hct of transfused blood (65\%)}}$$

The exchange is done over a 4- to 6-hour period, carefully following calcium, glucose, and hematocrit changes to avoid any metabolic or hemodynamic compromise from the massive blood exchange. Patients with recurrent acute chest syndromes are often on chronic simple transfusion therapy.

Other Issues

Children in the PICU need to be able to behave as a child as their medical condition allows. Physical, occupational, and play therapies are important parts of the medical care of a child. Physical therapists exercise the arms and legs of immobile patients, and occupational therapists place splints to prevent contractures. Children less ill often are able to color, play games, and enjoy videos. The spirit and mental health of a patient needs attention as does the body to insure that a mentally and physically healthy child leaves the PICU.

After the patient's medical needs have been attended to, the psychosocial issues should be addressed. Having a child in the PICU is a frightening and stressful situation and family members should be updated on a regular basis with all available information. Many families who have a child ill in the PICU find that the stress creates disruptions in the rest of their lives and, unfortunately, some couples experience irreconcilable differences during this period that later ends in divorce. Thus, it is very important for physicians to spend time talking with family members and attempt to answer any questions. If the child is medically stable and old enough to understand their illness, they should be included in discussions about their illness as well. Many children experiencing major illnesses in their young lives are wise and understand their conditions.

3

Neurocritical Care

Adnan I. Qureshi, Anish Bhardwaj, John A. Ulatowski

Advances in the diagnosis and treatment of neurological disease recently have led to a dramatic increase in neurocritical care units (NCCU). As most patients with life-threatening neurological diseases have systemic disease, the critical care unit facilitates an interdisciplinary approach to patient care that involves neurology, neurosurgery, anesthesiology, and internal medicine. Patients should receive neurocritical care if they have signs of raised intracranial pressure, coma, or neurological disease associated with respiratory or cardiovascular failure. Also, patients with subarachnoid hemorrhage or stroke, meningitis, encephalitis, status epilepticus, progressive muscular weakness, and head trauma may benefit from neurocritical care. Patients receiving thrombolytic therapy and plasmapheresis or those undergoing interventional neuroradiological procedures may benefit from neurocritical care as well.

NEUROLOGICAL EXAMINATION

An important part of the neurological examination in the NCCU is the assessment of level of consciousness. The neural tracts that mediate consciousness start from central pons and hypothalamus and project signals to the thalamus and cortex. Thalamic relay nuclei send diffuse projections to the cortex. The cortex feeds back on the thalamic nuclei promoting arousal. A depressed level of consciousness can occur from dysfunction of brainstem activating systems or impaired cerebral hemispheres, or both. Prior to assessment of consciousness, timing and dosing of administration of any sedative medication should be noted. The examination in the NCCU should consist of the following components:

Higher cortical functions:	Glasgow Coma Score
	Orientation and attention
	Speech
Cranial nerves and brainstem:	Midbrain-CN II: pupils, visual fields
	Midbrain-Pons-CN III, IV, VI: eye movements
	Pons-CN V: corneal reflex, facial sensation
	Lower Pons-CN VII: facial grimace and movements
	Lower Pons-CNVIII: oculocephalic/oculovestibular reflexes
	Medulla-CN IX,X: gag and cough reflex
	Medulla-CN XI: shoulder shrug
	Medulla-CN XII: tongue movements
Motor system:	Strength
	Tone
	Reflexes
	Plantar reflexes
Sensory system:	Pinprick perception
Cerebellar system:	Finger to nose testing
Meninges:	Neck rigidity

A detailed description of the important components is provided.

Higher Cortical Functions

Glasgow Coma Score (GCS)

GCS is a standard method of evaluating the level of consciousness and has demonstrated a high level of interobserver reliability. As shown in Table 3.1, GSC has three components—motor, eye, and verbal—which cannot be tested adequately in intubated patients. Further cortical functions including orientation, attention span, and speech (comprehension, expression, repetition, and naming) should be tested when possible.

Cranial Nerves and Brainstem

Pupillary Responses

The size of the pupils and, in particular, any asymmetry is noted. The response to light is assessed separately for both eyes using a

Table 3.1
Glasgow Coma Score

Best verbal response
1. No response
2. Incomprehensible sounds
3. Inappropriate words
4. Disoriented and converses
5. Fully oriented and converses

Best eye response
1. Does not open eyes
2. Opens eyes to painful stimuli
3. Opens eyes to verbal command
4. Opens eyes spontaneously

Best motor response
1. No motor response
2. Extension (decerebrate posturing)
3. Flexion (decorticate posturing)
4. Withdraws purposefully from painful stimuli
5. Localizes painful stimuli
6. Follows verbal commands

strong penlight, preferably in a dark room. The oculomotor nerve mediates the efferent limb of the pupillary response, causing pupillary constriction. Ipsilateral dilatation of the pupil with loss of pupillary reflex can signify transtentorial herniation, isolated third nerve palsy, or midbrain dysfunction.

Corneal Reflexes

The sensory component of the reflex is mediated by the trigeminal nerve, and the motor component by the facial nerve. The reflex is tested by bringing a wisp of cotton from the side, away from the visual fields. The sclera is touched gently and assessed for eyelid closure. The response is graded as absent, sluggish, and present. Bilateral loss of corneal reflexes is reflective of a poor level of consciousness. Unilateral loss is seen in lesions involving the trigeminal or facial nerve.

Eye Movements

First, notice the resting position of the eyes. The eyes are either midline or deviated toward one side (gaze deviation). Furthermore, the eyes can be conjugate (aligned together) or disconjugate (looking in separate directions). Eye movements can be observed by calling the attention of patient from one side and then the other or by attracting their attention with visual stimulus. However, in deeply comatose patients, it is not possible to observe eye movements in response to verbal stimuli. Oculocephalic reflex (OCR) is another method of testing eye movements and level of consciousness. The position of the eyes is recorded, and the head is turned toward one side (this maneuver should not be performed in patients with suspected cervical fracture). If the brainstem reflexes are intact, the eyes do not move with the head and remain fixated at primary gaze position. If the reflex is abolished, the eyes will move with the head. The OCR represents the brainstem mediated reflex that enables individuals to visually fixate on objects subconsciously while the head is moving. Oculovestibular reflex is another method of assessing the function of the brainstem. The head is elevated to an angle of 30°, 60 mL of cold water is instilled into one external ear, and the position of the eyes is recorded. The normal response is for the eyes to move toward the ear where the cold water is instilled. This response may take up to a minute. Testing of oculovestibular reflexes in each ear should be separated by at least two minutes to avoid contamination of the results.

Facial Grimace

In response to noxious stimuli, including intranares stimulation, the facial muscles contract. During contraction of the facial muscles, it is possible to detect any asymmetry in facial muscles or the facial nerve function.

Gag Reflex

The sensory component of this reflex is the glossopharyngeal (IX) nerve, and the motor component is mediated by the vagal nerve (X). The gag reflex can be tested by touching the posterior part of the oropharynx with a cotton tip and depressing the tongue to visually assess the contraction of the oropharynx. The gag reflex is a good test for evaluating the level of consciousness and the function of lower brainstem where the vagal and glossopharyngeal nerves originate.

Cough Reflex

The sensory and the motor component of this reflex is mediated through the vagas nerve. In intubated patients, a soft suction catheter is advanced through the endotracheal tube. A cough is the normal response, which is lost in comatose patients and patients with a brainstem lesion. The cough reflex is usually the last preserved reflex in a deteriorating level of consciousness.

Motor System

Muscle strength should be tested in proximal and distal muscles in each limb. In patients who are unable to follow commands, a standard noxious stimulus is applied to the sternum, stylomastoid process, or the supraorbital ridge, and the movement elicited in each limb is observed. Asymmetry can be detected in the movement elicited on both sides and usually suggests a focal lesion. A strong pinch is applied on each extremity (proximal and distal) and the response is graded as purposeful flexion, semipurposeful flexion, extension or posturing, and no response. It is important to note asymmetry in tone, bulk, and reflexes in each extremity to differentiate upper and lower motor neuron lesions. Presence of weakness with increased muscle tone, hyperreflexia, and extensor plantar response suggests an upper motor neuron lesion that can occur at any point in the corticospinal tract, including the motor cortex, brainstem, and spinal cord. It is important to recognize that the changes in tone and reflexes after upper motor lesion develop over days, and it is not unusual to see flaccidity and hyporeflexic extremities in the acute phase. Presence of extensor plantar response can be elicited by scratching the bottom of the foot looking for extension movement of the toes.

Sensory Examination

In patients unable to follow verbal commands, a limited sensory examination is performed that includes applying a noxious stimuli to each limb and observing for asymmetric facial grimace and limb withdrawal. In patients with intact level of consciousness, more detailed sensory testing should be performed. Recognizing sensory deficits helps in differentiating pure motor lesions from sensory motor lesions, which have different localization in the central nervous system. Determining a sensory level in patients helps localize lesions to the spinal cord.

Cerebellar Examination

Cerebellar functions should be assessed in each patient when possible. Finger to nose testing, touching the examiner's finger and subject's nose alternatively with the index finger, can help identify ipsilateral cerebellar ataxia.

Many neurological diseases are associated with abnormalities in respiration and hemodynamic status. Therefore, each neurological examination in the neurocritical care unit should evaluate respiration, blood pressure, and heart rate. The multiple patterns of respiration that can be observed in neurological disease include:

1. Hypoventilation consisting of shallow, rapid respirations in patients with a decreased level of consciousness or neuromuscular disease
2. Cheyne-Stokes breathing consisting of a regular waxing and waning respiration pattern. Cheyne-Stokes breathing is attributed to a decreased responsiveness of CO_2 receptors in the respiratory centers leading to retention of CO_2 followed by rapid respirations to reduce the CO_2. The respirations decrease after CO_2 is reduced and an alternating pattern of hyperventilation and hypoventilation is observed. This pattern is commonly seen in bilateral cortical damage.
3. Apnea described as episodes of absent respirations seen in infratentorial (brainstem or cerebellar) lesions. It is considered secondary to compression of respiratory centers in the lower brainstem.
4. Central hyperventilation consisting of very regular rapid respirations seen in high brainstem lesions

Airway protection is another major issue as a result of impaired oropharyngeal reflexes associated with a decreasing level of consciousness. Respiratory distress may be secondary to superimposed aspiration. For neurologic indications, securing the airway with an endotracheal tube may be necessary. Pulse oximeter monitoring is mandatory in every patient to assess the adequacy of the cardiopulmonary system as manifested by oxygen saturation.

Tachycardia or bradycardia can be the manifestations of acute intracranial process. Supraventricular tachycardias are the most common rhythm disturbances observed in patients with intracranial processes. Careful attention should be paid to the neurological status in patients in the neurocritical unit who present with new onset heart rate abnormalities. Other etiologies for tachycardias that should be considered are pain, anxiety or agitation, fever, hypoxemia, and volume depletion. Patients in the NCCU are monitored continuously using an electrocardiographic monitor. ECG changes in conduction, and axis deviation and repolarization occur frequently in patients with CNS disease but does not necessarily indicate coronary ischemia.

Blood pressure changes are common in the NCCU. Acute hypertension is seen with cerebral ischemia and raised intracranial pressure. It is important to recognize that hypertension represents a protective response to maintain cerebral perfusion in these conditions and should not be treated rapidly into the normal range. Other causes of hypertension include pain, agitation, or aggressive expression of previous hypertension (as a result of change in medications and high sympathetic activation). Hypotension is seen in patients with massive intracranial process and spinal cord injury because of loss of sympathetic tone and peripheral vasodilation. However, attempts should be made to evaluate for other causes of systemic hypotension including sepsis, fluid depletion, and effect of sedatives.

BASIC PATHOPHYSIOLOGIC PRINCIPLES

Mass Effect and Cerebral Herniations

The cranium represents a closed compartment. About 80% of the cranium's volume is occupied by the brain, 10% by the cerebrospinal fluid (CSF), and 10% by blood. Because of lack of expansible properties, small increases in the volume can lead to large increases in intracranial pressure (ICP). Initial increase in mass effect in any compartment is compensated by displacement of CSF leading to obliteration of sulci and ventricles. Further increase in volume in one compartment will push the normal contents into the other compartments within the cranium, a phenomenon known as herniation.

Subfalcine Herniation

Increase in mass effect in one hemisphere pushes the cingulate gyrus and the anterior cerebral artery to the other side under the falx (a vertical fibrous sheet that separates the upper part of both hemispheres). Patients usually present with a decreased level of consciousness and, sometimes, unilateral or bilateral anterior cerebral artery infarction with prominent leg weakness.

Transtentorial Herniation

A large increase in mass effect can lead to a downward shift of the hemisphere through the tentorium (a crescent shaped fibrous sheet that separates the hemispheres from the cerebellum). The uncus is the part of the hemisphere that herniates initially and compresses the ipsilateral third nerve leading to pupillary dilatation (uncal herniation). Further expansion compresses the corticospinal tracts leading to contralateral hemiparesis.

Central Herniation

Bilateral vertical shift (hydrocephalus) or diffuse parenchymal swelling can lead to herniation of both hemispheres causing bilateral pupillary dilatation, loss of consciousness, and quadriparesis.

Transforaminal Herniation

Increase in mass effect in the brainstem and cerebellar region can lead to protrusion of the cerebellar tonsils through the foramen magnum. Initial presentation includes apnea and cardiovascular compromise as a result of direct compression of respiratory and cardiovascular centers in the medulla.

Cerebral Edema

Cerebral edema represents an important component of mass effect from any cerebral lesion. The three types of cerebral edema are as follows:

Vasogenic Edema

This represents excess extracellular fluid in the brain as a result of a breakdown of the blood-brain barrier. This form of edema is seen with tumors and abscesses and is responsive to steroid treatment.

Cytotoxic Edema

Owing to direct cellular damage, the transport system of the cell membrane is impaired leading to accumulation of water within the cells. This type of edema is seen in cerebral infarction and is not responsive to steroid treatment. The edema observed in traumatic injury and intracranial hemorrhage represents a combination of both cytotoxic and vasogenic edema.

Interstitial Edema

Extravasation of fluid through the ventricular ependymal layering as a result of hydrocephalus can lead to accumulation of fluid in the periventricular spaces. This type of edema has minimal mass effect and responds to ventricular drainage.

Intracranial Pressure

Intracranial pressure (ICP) is the pressure within the cranial vault. Normal value is 5 to 15 mm Hg (10 to 20 cm of H_2O). ICP greater than 20 mm Hg is taken as the threshold for starting treatment to reduce ICP. The ICP can be measured in the subarachnoid space, ventricular cavity, and the brain parenchyma by using a subarachnoid bolt, ventricular catheter, and Camino monitor respectively. A subarachnoid bolt is a small catheter that is placed through the cranium into the subarachnoid space over the frontal lobe and then connected to a transducer. A ventricular catheter is placed in the lateral ventricle through the cranium, frontal lobe, and into the frontal horn of the lateral ventricle. The catheter is capable of measuring ICP as well as drainage of CSF. The Camino device is a fiberoptic device that is placed over the brain parenchyma to measure parenchymal pressure.

Cerebral Perfusion Pressure (CPP)

CPP is a derived measure representative of cerebral blood flow (CBF). It is function of both systemic blood pressure and intracranial pressure and is estimated as CPP = MAP (mean arterial pressure) − ICP. Although an indirect measure of CBF, CPP should be kept above 70 mm Hg. The cerebral arterioles maintain constant blood flow by altering their diameter with changing systemic MAP, a phenomenon known as autoregulation. Under normal autoregulation, both CPP and CBF are preserved within systemic MAP range of 60 to 150 mm Hg. However, conditions that elevate ICP usually impair the normal autoregulatory capacity. Therefore, maintaining adequate perfusion pressure requires reduction of ICP and, at times, augmentation of systemic blood pressure.

BASIC TREATMENT PRINCIPLES

Treatment of Raised ICP

The following treatment modalities are available for management of raised intracranial pressure:

Hyperventilation

Artificial hyperventilation to reduce $PaCO_2$ to 25 to 30 mm Hg is used for acute treatment of raised ICP. Lowering the $PaCO_2$ induces local alkalosis in the extracellular spaces of cerebral tissue leading to vasoconstriction of the cerebral arterioles. This reduces the blood volume in the cranial vault and reduces the ICP. The effect is transient (6 to 24 hours) and, therefore, hyperventilation should be used only for acute emergent situations and not prophylactically. The potential for inducing cerebral ischemia with hyperventilation has been described previously.

Mannitol

Mannitol is an osmotic agent that reduces the cerebral water content and therefore reduces ICP. Furthermore, mannitol increases the viscosity of blood in the cerebral arterioles and induces vasoconstriction leading to reduction in ICP. The initial dose is 0.5 g/kg and the maintenance dose is 0.25 g/kg every 4 to 6 hours to keep serum osmolality between 310 and 320 mOsm/L. Serum osmolality must be monitored frequently when repeated doses of mannitol are used.

CSF Drainage

ICP is reduced by decreasing the ventricular volume in cases of hydrocephalus. CSF drainage from the ventricular cavities creates a gradient for movement of extracellular fluid from the edematous regions into the ventricles and subsequent drainage.

Pentobarbital

Pentobarbital reduces the cerebral metabolism, cerebral blood flow volume, and consequently, the ICP. The induction dose is 40 mg/kg intravenous bolus over 4 hours and maintenance dose is 1 to 2 mg/kg per hour. The cerebral activity is monitored by continuous electroencephalography (EEG), and the goal is to induce burst suppression where there is occasional spontaneous electrical activity followed by suppression of baseline EEG rhythm. Pentobarbital is a cardiovascular and respiratory depressant that requires intensive cardiovascular monitoring with a pulmonary artery catheter and mechanical ventilation. Pentobarbital also reduces gastric motility and impairs immune function. As a result of the complications associated with a pentobarbital coma and uncertain outcome efficacy, pentobarbital should be used only in cases with ICP resistant to standard therapy.

Steroids

Steroids reduce vasogenic edema and therefore reduce ICP. However, steroids have only demonstrated benefit in vasogenic edema owing to neoplasm and have a long onset of action; therefore, they have a limited use in acute management of raised ICP.

Mechanical Ventilation

Three important reasons for intubation and mechanical ventilation in the neurointensive care unit are as follows.

1. *Airway protection as a result of poor level of consciousness.* These patients do well on synchronized intermittent mechanical ventilation (SIMV) or continuous pressure support if their respiratory drives are intact. As the level of consciousness improves, the patients can be placed directly on IMV rate of 2 or continuous pressure support (CPAP). Serial assessment of the level of consciousness and cough reflex can provide a useful index for planning extubation. If the patient's level of consciousness fails to improve in two weeks, or they demonstrate poor airway protection after extubation, the patient undergoes tracheostomy.
2. *Decreased or absent ventilatory drive as a result of brainstem lesions.*

These patients usually have concomitant impairment of airway protective reflexes as well, and can be maintained on SIMV. In the absence of any improvement, these patients require tracheostomy and chronic mechanical ventilation.

3. *Decreased ventilatory strength as a result of neuromuscular disease.* CO_2 retention and patient comfort are the best guide of adequacy of ventilatory support. End tidal CO_2 can be monitored using capnography attached to the ventilator. In the acute phase of the disease, these patients are most comfortable on assist control (AC) mechanical ventilation, because they get support with every breath taken and can adjust their respiratory rate according to need. Patients with reversible neuromuscular conditions, such as Guillain-Barré syndrome and myasthenia gravis, can be weaned from ventilation. The duration of weaning is variable depending on the individual's general health and severity of the disease. Forced vital capacity and negative inspiratory force are measured daily to quantitate progress and guide the weaning process.

Blood Pressure (BP) Management

The goal of BP management is to maintain adequate cerebral perfusion. The MAP goal in the neurocritical unit is usually higher than required for systemic perfusion. The goal is to maintain adequate cerebral perfusion. The lower limit of blood pressure should be adequate to keep CPP greater than 70 mm Hg. In the absence of high ICP, MAP of 90 or greater should be adequate for maintaining cerebral blood flow. Any hypotension should be treated aggressively. Intravenous fluids and phenylephrine or dopamine can be used to increase systemic blood pressure.

Acute hypertension in patients with intracranial disease can be a protective response to either raised intracranial pressure or cerebral ischemia. Lowering blood pressure in such situations can worsen cerebral perfusion. If blood pressure has to be reduced, thiopental (a short-acting barbiturate) in doses of 100 to 200 mg intravenously is a good choice because it reduces cerebral metabolism and ICP and lowers blood pressure, thus protecting against cerebral hypoperfusion. Another important cause of acute hypertension is agitation which responds to sedation.

Choosing which antihypertensive to use is also important. Nitrates and nitroprusside, which usually are avoided, can lead to cerebral vasodilation and increase the ICP. Sublingual nifedipine can lower the blood pressure precipitously and cause cerebral ischemia and is avoided. Labetalol is an alpha and beta antagonist used as a first-line antihypertensive which has little effect on cerebral vasculature. An initial dose of 5 mg intravenously is used as a test dose, as some patients may have a precipitous drop of BP, especially if they are dehydrated. After the first dose, 10 to 40 mg intravenously every 10 to 15 minutes can be used to reduce blood pressure to desirable goals. Bradycardia prior to antihypertensive effect may require another agent. Intravenous hydralazine, which is a direct acting vasodilator, can be used in doses of 10 to 20 mg every 15 minutes. Another intravenous agent with little effect on cerebral vasculature is enalapril (an angiotensin converting enzyme inhibitor), which is used in doses of 1.25 to 2.5 mg every 6 hours.

Fluid Status Management

The optimal fluid status for most patients with neurological disease is euvolemia. Systemic dehydration does not reduce cerebral edema but may worsen cerebral perfusion. Therefore, adequate fluid intake should be provided for all patients. In healthy adults, sufficient fluid is required to balance gastrointestinal losses of 100 to 200 mL/day, insensible losses of 500 to 1000 mL/day through cutaneous and respiratory route, and urinary losses of 1000 mL/day. Average maintenance fluid is approximately 2000 to 2500 mL/day for adults. Most patients require a greater amount of fluids in the ICU because of large losses during tachypnea, fever, and use of osmotic agents. Normal saline is the intravenous fluid of choice. Hypotonic solutions can worsen cerebral edema and are avoided. Glucose-containing solutions, which are avoided as well, can worsen cerebral injury as ischemic neural tissue metabolizes glucose to lactic acid by anaerobic metabolism.

Nutrition

Metabolic activity is increased in many neurological diseases such as head trauma and spinal injury. Therefore, nutrition intake should be started as soon as possible to avoid a negative nitrogen balance. Because of a decreased level of consciousness, most patients require a nasogastric tube for administration of nutritional preparations. Ileus and delayed gastric emptying are common occurrences in the NCCU. Metoclopramide (Reglan) intravenously 10 mg every 4 hours may be required for large gastric residuals. Both head or spine trauma result in constipation requiring laxatives. Gastrointestinal motility is also worsened by narcotics, barbiturates, and systemic infections. Sometimes intravenous nutrition may be required.

Sedation

Sedation is required for patients who are confused and agitated, are in discomfort because of pain or endotracheal tube intubation, or are manifesting hyperadrenergic symptoms as a result of drug or alcohol withdrawal. The sedation regimen should preserve the neurological examination as required for constant neurological monitoring, or have the potential to be discontinued with rapid return of an uncompromised examination. Increasing confusion and agitation may be manifestations of increasing ICP or a new cerebral lesion, therefore, a careful assessment prior to administration of any sedation is required. The four most common agents used in the ICU are benzodiazepines, narcotics, haloperidol, and propofol. Midalozam is a short-acting benzodiazepine used in bolus doses of 0.02 to 0.08 mg/kg or as an infusion at 0.05 to 0.1 mg/kg per hour. Midalozam reduces the cerebral metabolism without significantly altering the cerebral blood flow and can be used for infusions lasting less than 24 hours. Fentanyl is a synthetic opiate with rapid distribution and short half-life. The usual dose for bolus is 0.25 to 1.5 μg/kg and infusion is 0.3 to 1.5 μg/kg per hour. Major side effects include respiratory depression and hypotension. Naloxone, if required, is used to reverse the adverse effects of opiates. Haloperidol is a butyrophenone that has minimal effect on respiratory and cardiovascular status. The usual dose is 0.01 to 0.05 mg/kg. Propofol is an ultrashort-acting alkyl phenol. Its clinical action on cerebral activity and intracranial dynamics is similar to short-acting barbiturates. The usual dose is 0.3 to 2.0 mg/kg for boluses and 0.6 to 6.0 mg/kg per hour for infusion. The main side effects include respiratory depression and hypotension. Propofol is used only in intubated patients.

Head Trauma

The primary injury in head trauma is hemorrhagic with extradural, subdural, or parenchymal involvement; and a nonhemorrhagic component consists of cellular swelling, vasogenic edema, and contusions and diffuse axonal injury. Diffuse axonal injury results from the shear stress induced by rapid acceleration/deceleration of the neural tissue. In its severe form, hemorrhagic foci in the corpus callosum and dorsolateral rostral brainstem with microscopic evidence of diffuse injury to the axons (axonal retraction balls, microglial stars, and degeneration of white matter tracts) are observed. Diffuse axonal injury can present as protracted loss of consciousness immediately after head trauma in the absence of any mass occupying lesions on CT scan. Secondary injury commonly results from hypotension or hypoxia. Management of head trauma is based on the following principles:

Support vital signs by managing the airway and normalizing blood pressure and heart rhythm. Patients with GCS of 8 or below should be intubated.

The paO_2 should be maintained above 100 mm Hg and the initial MAP goal is 90 mm Hg or above. Once ICP recordings are available, the CPP should be kept above 70 mm Hg. Intravenous fluids and vasopressors may be required to support blood pressure.

An ICP monitor, preferably a ventriculostomy, should be placed in patients with GCS of 8 or less to guide treatment. Hyperventilation is used to reduce $PaCO_2$ to 25 to 30 mm Hg if evidence is clear of increased ICP either on the basis of ICP monitors recordings or clinical examination including unilateral or bilateral pupillary dilatation with loss of light reflex and decreased level of consciousness. Mannitol therapy should be initiated concomitantly. Hyperventilation is then weaned and, in the absence of high ICP, $PaCO_2$ is kept between 30 and 35 mm Hg.

Surgical evacuation of extradural, subdural or intracerebral hematomas is considered. The size of the lesion and the clinical status determine eligibility for surgical evacuation.

Anticonvulsants should be started on a prophylactic basis. Phenytoin and carbamazepine have demonstrated efficacy in preventing acute posttraumatic seizures. Phenytoin (20 mg/kg) is loaded intravenously at a rate less than 50 mg/min and then 100 mg every 8 hours for maintenance. Steroids have no demonstrated efficacy in head trauma and are avoided.

The ICP rise is most prominent on day 3 because of coalescence of small hemorrhages and worsening cerebral edema. ICP greater than 20 mm Hg should be treated with mannitol. If ICP does not respond to repeated doses of mannitol or serum osmolality greater than 310 mOsm/L, then either pentobarbital coma or decompressive surgery should be considered. Factors that exacerbate ICP, such as fever, agitation, and high $PaCO_2$, are aggressively treated. A second rise in ICP is seen in some patients at day 10, again, requiring standard ICP treatment.

At 2 weeks, if patients are unable to protect their airway because of poor functional outcome, tracheostomy and percutaneous gastrostomy tube placement are considered in preparation for subacute or chronic care.

INTRACEREBRAL HEMORRHAGE (ICH)

Nontraumatic intracerebral hemorrhage can present with acute onset of loss of consciousness and focal deficits. Most spontaneous ICH are the result of underlying hypertension. The diagnosis is made on CT scan. The management principles are described.

Airway Support

Patients with GCS of 8 or less usually are intubated.

Blood Pressure Control

Most patients are hypertensive at presentation as a consequence of preexisting hypertension and raised intracranial pressure. Hematomas continue to expand in the first few hours after onset in many patients. High blood pressure may predispose to expansion of hematomas. Blood pressure is reduced if MAP is greater than 140 to 150 mm Hg for more than 15 minutes, according to the recommendations of National Stroke Association. However, blood pressure should not be treated aggressively particularly in the absence of knowledge regarding ICP. The hematoma induces a zone of ischemia around itself by compression of microvasculature in the surrounding tissue. Lowering the blood pressure precipitously can worsen tissue damage as a result of ischemia.

A coagulation profile is performed, which includes prothrombin time, activated partial thromboplastin time, and platelet count. Patients who have an abnormal coagulation profile may require fresh frozen plasma or platelet replacement to prevent expansion of hematoma.

Patients who have blood in the ventricles are at risk for developing obstructive hydrocephalus as the blood clot prevents drainage of CSF. A ventricular catheter is inserted in patients with hydrocephalus.

Evacuation of the clot is recommended if cerebellar hemorrhages threaten transforaminal herniation and compression of medulla. Evacuation of the hematoma in other sites depends on the clinical condition and size of the clot.

Most patients have preexisting hypertension. Oral hypertensive should be held in the first 48 hours because of long half-lives and unpredictable response in the presence of elevated ICP. Blood pressure should be managed by intravenous antihypertensive with shorter half-lives and titrated to response. Oral antihypertensives can be started after 48 hours if the patient's condition is stabilizing.

Elevated ICP can be seen in ICH and is a result of mass effect of the hematoma and cerebral edema around the hematoma. Cerebral edema is maximum at 48 hours and starts to recede after 5 days. Standard measures of ICP control may be required.

Some patients have a poor recovery and will require a tracheostomy and a gastric tube for supportive care. Patients who have a poor level of consciousness at presentation and have a large hematoma on CT scan usually have a poor recovery.

SUBARACHNOID HEMORRHAGE

Subarachnoid hemorrhage (SAH) is a blood clot in the subarachnoid space prominent at the base of the brain. Most subarachnoid hemorrhages are the result of a ruptured cerebral aneurysm. The diagnosis is made on the CT scan. In cases where clinical picture is very suggestive of SAH and the CT scan is negative (10%), a lumbar puncture is performed to look for blood and xanthochromia (color due to breakdown products of bilirubin) in the CSF. Once the diagnosis is established, the following management is recommended:

A four-vessel cerebral angiography is performed as early as possible to diagnose the aneurysm. About 20% of patients may have multiple aneurysms. Surgical clipping of the aneurysm is performed early to prevent rebleeding. Aggressive control of the BP is needed to avoid rebleeding of the aneurysm, keeping in mind the CPP goals. Control of headache with acetaminophen/ or narcotics is recommended. Anxious patients are sedated with low-dose phenobarbital (30 mg po every 6 to 8 hours). Nimodipine (60 mg po every 4 hours) and anticonvulsant are initiated for prophylaxis of cerebral, vasospasm, and seizures respectively. Some physicians use steroids (decadron 4 mg every 6 hours) to reduce chemical meningitis associated with subarachnoid hemorrhage.

Patients are at risk for cerebral vasospasm after SAH, because oxyhemoglobin released from the breakdown of the clot induces constriction of the cerebral blood vessels. The reduction in CBF as a result of vasospasm is compensated by collateral circulation. Cerebral vasospasm occurs in two-thirds of the patients 3 to10 days after SAH. Cerebral ischemia (clinical vasospasm) is seen in only half of patients with vasospasm that may manifest as focal deficit, decreased level of consciousness, or a combination. The onset can be acute or insidious over 24 hours. Daily TCD ultrasound is performed for early detection of cerebral vasospasm. This noninvasive test measures the velocity of cerebral blood flow. Increased velocities signify cerebral vasospasm. Once the aneurysm is secured, modest hypervolemia (central venous pressure [CVP] of 5 to 8 mm Hg) is maintained to prevent cerebral ischemia from vasospasm. If cerebral ischemia occurs as a result of vasospasm, hypervolemia and hypertension are instituted. Hypervolemia (CVP of 8 to 12 mm Hg or pulmonary capillary wedge pressure of 12 to 14 mm Hg) is achieved by intravenously administering normal saline at a rate of 150 to 200 mL/hour, however, intermittent bolus of normal saline or colloids may be required. Hypertension is achieved by administering phenylephrine or ionotropic infusion to increase the mean arterial pressure (100 to 140 mm Hg) and cardiac output. If there is no response within 4 hours, therapies such as intra-arterial papaverine or angioplasty are considered. Once the clinical symptoms have improved, the hypertensive/hypervolemic therapy is weaned titrated over 48 hours under close observation for recurrence of cerebral ischemia.

Obstructive hydrocephalus can result from blood in the ventricles or subarachnoid blood obstructing the arachnoid villi (where CSF is absorbed into the venous sinuses). The symptom consists of a decreased level of consciousness. Immediate treatment is insertion of a ventricular catheter. The blood dissolves over time, and the hydrocephalus can resolve. However, sometimes, fibrosis develops within the arachnoid villi and a ventriculoperitoneal shunt may be required for chronic CSF diversion.

Any neurologic deterioration is investigated aggressively by a CT scan to rule out hydrocephalus. CSF and serum analysis is performed to rule out meningitis and electrolyte disturbances respectively. A cerebral angiography may be required to diagnose vasospasm.

Steroids, if used, are quickly tapered over a few days. By the end of the second week, hypervolemic therapy is titrated against TCD velocities and neurologic examination. Nimodipine is continued for 21 days after onset of SAH.

CEREBRAL INFARCTION

Cerebral infarction results from thrombotic or embolic occlusion of an artery supplying the brain. Emboli can originate from a proximal artery (such as an atherosclerotic plague in the carotid artery or aorta), cardiac valves, or left ventricle. Middle cerebral artery (MCA) infarction consists of hemiparesis, hemisensory loss, aphasia or neglect, and gaze deviation. Vertebrobasilar artery infarction presents as a combination of a decreased level of consciousness, cranial nerve involvement, and cerebellar dysfunction. Infarction may not be visualized on CT scan up to 24 hours, therefore, diagnosis is made clinically on most occasions or by magnetic resonance imaging. Management is based on the following principles:

Airway Management

Patients with vertebrobasilar ischemia are at risk for respiratory compromise because of a decreased level of consciousness, central apnea, and poor airway protective reflexes. Intubation is considered early. Patients with MCA infarction develop decreased level of consciousness when cerebral edema is maximum (2 to 5 days after onset) and may require intubation at that point.

Blood Pressure Management

Elevated BP in cerebral infarction is a response to preserve cerebral blood flow. Blood pressure should only be reduced if it is greater than 220/120 for over 15 minutes according to the recommendations of the National Stroke Association. Aggressive lowering of BP is avoided unless signs of hypertensive encephalopathy develop. Oral antihypertensive agents should be started at the end of the first week.

Tissue Plasminogen Activator Administration

Intravenous tissue plasminogen activator (tPA) administration improves outcome if given within 3 hours of symptom onset. Theoretically, the tPA lyses the clot and restores blood flow in the affected distribution. The dose is 0.9 mg/kg, of which 10% is given as a bolus followed by an infusion over 1 hour. The greatest risk with tPA is hemorrhagic transformation. After the lysis of the clot, the blood flow returns and enters the parenchyma through the disrupted blood-brain barrier. To avoid the risk of hemorrhagic transformation, the CT scan should not show evidence of large cerebral infarction prior to administration of tPA.

Present studies have shown that there is viable tissue within the periphery of ischemic zone. This tissue is partially ischemic and is very sensitive to potential secondary neuronal injuries such as hyperglycemia and hyperpyrexia. Therefore, strict glucose and temperature control should be instituted in the acute phase of infarction.

Intravenous heparin is given in acute cerebral infarction for either preventing extension of the clot and progression of deficits or reducing the risk of further embolization from a cardiac source. Patients with atrial fibrillation and dilated cardiomyopathy should be considered for acute anticoagulation because of the high risk of recurrent embolization. Because of the high risk of hemorrhagic transformation with heparin, most physicians would wait 48 hours and repeat the CT scan. If there is no evidence of hemorrhagic transformation, intravenous heparin is started. Boluses of heparin should be avoided. Vertebrobasilar artery infarction is another reasonable indication for intravenous heparin, and the deficits can progress in 40% of the patients; therefore, heparin without a bolus dose is started at presentation in such patients. The goal of intravenous heparin treatment is a PTT of 1.5 to 1.8 times control and infusion usually is continued for 4 days. Thereafter, patients are put on coumadin or aspirin depending on the etiology of infarction. Patients who are not anticoagulation candidates should be started on aspirin (325 mg/day) on presentation.

Cerebral edema seen in cerebral infarction is predominantly cytotoxic with a less prominent vasogenic component. It peaks at 48 hours and starts resolving by 5 days. Cerebral edema can cause life-threatening mass effect (herniation). Decompression of the infarcted tissue may be necessary. Standard treatment for edema (hyperventilation, osmotic therapy) is instituted as indicated.

Echocardiography and cerebral angiography may be performed early to determine underlying etiology of cerebral infarction. Patients with a cardioembolic source would require long-term anticoagulation. Patients with vertebrobasilar atherosclerosis also are considered for long-term anticoagulation. Significant carotid stenosis, which is narrowing greater than 70% of unaffected segment, should be evaluated for carotid endarterectomy.

STATUS EPILEPTICUS

Status epilepticus is continuous or intermittent seizure activity without regaining consciousness for a period greater than 30 minutes. At present, most neurologists consider any seizure activity lasting more than 10 minutes as ominous and would start aggressive treatment. Initial treatment consists of intravenous administration of a benzodiazepine, such as lorazepam, in repeated doses of 1 mg every 5 minutes. Patients showing signs of respiratory depression are intubated. At the same time, intravenous phenytoin is administered in doses of 20 mg/kg at a rate no faster than 50 mg/min. If seizures continue, another 5 mg/kg of phenytoin can be given. If seizures are not responsive to aggressive phenytoin therapy, either a benzodiazepine (midazolam) infusion is started with a bolus of 0.2 mg/kg followed by an infusion of 0.1 to 0.4 mg/kg per hour; or intravenous phenobarbital in doses of 5 to 10 mg/kg is administered. Patients definitely require intubation at this point. Patients who still are unresponsive to treatment are placed into a pentobarbital coma. The loading dose is 12 mg/kg with a maintenance infusion of 5 mg/kg per hour. Patients who are in pentobarbital coma should be on a continuous EEG monitor to titrate to complete seizure control or burst suppression pattern if required.

Electrolyte abnormalities including glucose, calcium and magnesium can exacerbate seizures. Head CT is obtained in patients with new onset seizures. Lumbar puncture is considered if the head CT does not rule out infections. Seizures are prominent in herpes simplex encephalitis and bacterial meningitis.

The seizures stop in most patients with a combination of benzodiazepines and phenytoin. A period of unresponsiveness after cessation of seizures is not unusual as a result of postictal state and medication effect. If patients do not start improving over 6 to 8 hours, the following possibilities should be considered:

1. Continuing nonconvulsive status epilepticus, where the motor manifestations have stopped, but electrical activity is continuing within the brain
2. Hypoxic–ischemic damage sustained during convulsions
3. An underlying structural/metabolic abnormality

Complications of status epilepticus include hypoxic organ damage, aspiration of gastric contents, and rhabdomyolysis. Patients are hydrated and creatine phosphokinase levels and renal functions are monitored. Hyperpyrexia is not unusual because of excess muscle activity.

Most patients make good recovery from status epilepticus. Long-term anticonvulsants should be initiated early if indicated.

GUILLAIN-BARRÉ SYNDROME

Guillain-Barré syndrome (GBS) is a demyelinating disease of peripheral nerves that progresses over 2 weeks to maximum severity. Clinical presentation includes acute quadriparesis (more prominent in the lower extremities) with or without cranial nerve involvement. Diagnosis is made on the basis of clinical presentation and CSF analysis that reveals elevated protein in the absence of leukocytosis. Nerve conduction studies are helpful in diagnosing conduction block due to demyelination. Critical care issues include respiratory failure and autonomic dysfunction. The management is based on the following principles:

Respiratory Support

The decision to intubate is made on the basis of clinical evaluation that includes assessment of the strength of cough and sniff. Patients can be asked to count loudly as long as possible on one breath. Normal persons can count easily to 30, while patients who count to less than 20 have significant impairment of respiratory muscles. Forced vital capacity (FVC) and negative inspiratory force (NIF) is measured every 4 to 6 hours. Patients who have FVC < 15 mL/kg and NIF < 25 mm Hg usually are intubated. Because of concomitant facial weakness, it may be difficult to establish a tight seal on the mouth piece for such ventilatory parameters. Therefore, parameter results are interpreted in conjunction with clinical evaluation. Once the patient is intubated, full support is advised for the early part of mechanical ventilation. Assist control or IMV modes in the acute phase of the disease offer complete rest for the respiratory muscles. The adequacy of ventilatory support is determined by patient comfort and lack of CO_2 retention. After the acute phase, the patient can be placed on CPAP and pressure support can be titrated down as tolerated. Daily FVC and NIF are measured to follow improvement in respiratory muscle strength. Patients are likely to be extubated if FVC and NIF are greater than 15 mL/kg and 25 cm H_2O respectively.

Immunoglobulin or Plasma Exchange

Treatment of acute demyelination requires administration of either immunoglobulin or plasma exchange. Intravenous immunoglobulins are as effective as plasma exchange and are easier to administer and, therefore, should be used as the first line of treatment. The dose is 0.4 gm/kg per day for 5 days. Complications include renal impairment, aseptic meningitis, hay-fever-like syndrome and hyperviscosity syndrome. Plasma exchange is reserved for patients who fail to respond to immunoglobulin treatment or who relapse after initial improvement. Usually five plasma exchanges (each of 200 to 250 mL/kg) are performed.

Autonomic lability that includes tachycardia with occasional arrhythmias and blood pressure fluctuations can be observed in the acute period. The first choice should be to avoid pharmacological treatment because of the transient and unpredictable nature of these episodes. If symptoms necessitate treatment, standard short-acting cardiac medications are effective.

Treatment of Pain

Pain is an important component of GBS and usually is located in the back and shoulder regions worsening at night. Narcotics are used if required. Sometimes when constipation and urinary retention become an issue as a result of narcotic use and autonomic dysfunction, intravenous ketorolac can be used. Longer acting and less addictive medications, such as tricyclic antidepressants, nonsteroidal anti-inflammatory agents, and anticonvulsants, are used chronically with some effect.

MYASTHENIC CRISIS

Myasthenia gravis is a disease in which autoantibodies directed against the acetylcholine receptors at the neuromuscular junction lead to muscle weakness. Acute weakness of the respiratory and/or bulbar muscles due to myasthenia gravis is known as myasthenic crisis. It is usually precipitated by infections, initiation of steroids, or change in medication. Clinical presentation are of two types: 1) respiratory distress with excessive effort of the respiratory muscles; or 2) in severe muscle weakness, the patient is hypercarbic with poor effort and somnolescence. The management is based on the following principles:

Respiratory Support

The respiratory failure in myasthenic crisis does not improve quickly and the patients progressively get worse as a result of fatigue. Therefore, early intubation with mechanical support should be instituted early in the episode. Patients should be fully supported in the early part of mechanical ventilation; most physicians would use assist control or IMV in the acute phase of the disease to completely rest the respiratory muscles. The adequacy of ventilatory support is determined by patient comfort and lack of CO_2 retention. After the first two days, the patient can be placed on CPAP, and pressure support can be titrated down as tolerated. Daily FVC and NIF are measured to follow improvement in respiratory muscle strength. Patients are likely to be extubated if FVC and NIF are greater than 15 mL/kg and 25 cm H_20 respectively. Oropharyngeal secretions can be a problem as a result of the cholinergic effect of anticholinesterase agents used in the treatment of myasthenia. Oral glycopyrrolate (1mg every 6 hours) can be used to reduce these secretions. Patients are at risk to develop atelectasis because of poor inflation of the lungs and require sighs on the ventilator with postural drainage of the affected lungs if atelectases develops.

Plasmapheresis or Intravenous Immunoglobulin Administration

Treatment of myasthenia requires either plasmapheresis or intravenous immunoglobulin administration. Plasmapheresis removes the anticholinergic receptor antibodies in the serum and improves clinical symptoms. Usually five exchanges are performed on alternate days. Intravenous immunoglobulin can be used in patients if plasmapheresis is not feasible. Immunoglobulins reduce production of other immunoglobulins, such as anticholinergic antibodies, as a result of negative feedback. Also, immunoglobulins bind to antibodies neutralizing their antigen binding capacity. The usual dose is 0.4 gm/kg per day intravenously for 5 days.

Steroid Treatment

To improve acute symptoms of myasthenia, high-dose steroid treatment is used including methyl prednisone 100 mg every 8 hours or oral prednisone 80 mg a day for three days followed by a taper to maintenance dose.

Other measures include treatment of infections, and removal of medication that exacerbate myasthenia.

SPINAL CORD TRAUMA

Acute spinal cord injury has an initial component of contusion and intraparenchymal or extradural hemorrhage followed by release of prostaglandins from the breakdown of cellular membranes. These prostaglandin derivatives lead to vasoconstriction and secondary ischemia in the local tissue. The acute management is based on the following principles:

All patients who present within 8 hours of injury should receive a high-dose steroid (methylprednisolone), which includes a bolus dose of 30 mg/kg followed by an infusion of 5.4 mg/kg per hour for 23 hours. High-dose steroids reduce the release and activation of prostaglandin metabolites and, presumably, reduce secondary injury. Blood pressure usually is augmented using vasopressors to increase perfusion of the spinal cord for the first 24 hours.

Patients who have high cervical injury (damage to phrenic nerve) require mechanical ventilation if no other complications are present.

In the initial phase of spinal cord injury, vasodilation and hypotension occur owing to loss of sympathetic innervation. This is particularly prominent in lesions above the 6th thoracic level, because the innervation of the splanchnic vessels comes out at that level. Aggressive intravenous fluid and vasopressors may be required during this period to maintain adequate blood pressure. However, this vasodilatory phase is followed by increased sympathetic tone and vasoconstriction because of loss of higher control over a period of 48 to 72 hours. This period can be associated with autonomic dysfunction, such as a significant rise in blood pressure in response to sympathetic stimulation by pain, urinary bladder distension, or constipation. Intravenous vasodilators, general anaesthetics, or regional blockage of neural impulses with spinal or epidural anaesthesia may be necessary.

INFECTIONS OF THE CENTRAL NERVOUS SYSTEM

Bacterial Meningitis

Clinical presentation includes fever, headache, and neck rigidity. Diagnosis is established by CSF analysis. Most common organisms in adults include N. meningitidis, S. pneumoniae, and H. influenzae. The initial treatment is started with intravenous ceftriaxone 2 gm every 12 hours or cefotaxime 2 gm every 6 hours. In older adults (over 50 years), ampicillin (2 gm every 4 hours) is added to cover for S.agalactiae and Listeria monocytogenes. In patients with impaired cellular immunity, ampicillin and a broad spectrum cephalosporin such as ceftazidime is used for empiric therapy. In patients with recent head trauma or neurosurgery, administer broad spectrum antibiotics that are effective against both Gram-positive and Gram-negative, such as vancomycin and ceftazidime. If the Gram stain of the CSF is suggestive of S.pneumonia, a second agent such as vancomycin or rifampicin is added because of the high incidence of penicillin-resistant S.pneumonia. Treatment is continued until the organism in CSF is identified, and then antibiotics can be adjusted based on the antibiotic-susceptibility of the organism. If no clinical response is seen within 72 hours of initiating treatment, a repeat lumbar puncture is performed and antibiotics are changed. Some authorities advocate steroid use for reducing long-term effects of inflammation in the subarachnoid space, such as deafness and hydrocephalus in patients with a high concentration of bacteria in the CSF (bacteria visible on gram stain of CSF) and elevated ICP. Dexamethasone (0.15 mg/kg every 6 hours for 4 days) is the recommended treatment. The antibiotic treatment is continued for 10 to 14 days in S.pneumoniae meningitis and 7 days in H.influenzae or N.meningitidis meningitis. Infection with L.monocytogenes and Gram-negative bacilli should be treated for 14 to 21 days.

Viral Encephalitis

The clinical presentation includes fever, change in mental status, and seizures. Presence of focal deficits suggests herpes simplex encephalitis. The CSF profile consists of lymphocytosis with elevated protein and normal glucose. Magnetic resonance imaging can reveal diffuse involvement of the brain parenchyma, particularly the temporal lobes in HSV encephalitis. Intravenous acyclovir is started when there is a suspicion of encephalitis. The dose is 10 mg/kg every 8 hours, and treatment is continued for two weeks. The presence of HSV in the CSF is confirmed by polymerase chain reaction. Viral cultures take up to 2 weeks and have little impact on treatment. In case of acyclovir resistance, arabinoside and foscarnet are other antiviral agents to consider effective against HSV.

Cerebral Abscess

Clinical presentation includes fever, change in level of consciousness, and focal deficits. The diagnosis can be made on both CT scan or MRI. The most common organism is streptococcus pneumoniae. A superimposed anaerobic infection is in the necrotic abscess as well. The first line of treatment is intravenous antibiotics consisting of intravenous penicillin (4 million units every 4 hours) and metronidazole (500 mg every 6 hours) for 4 weeks. Surgical aspiration is avoided because of the risk of disseminating infection through the aspiration track. If clinical symptoms do not resolve after 1 week of treatment and the abscess is unchanged or larger on follow-up CT scan, then surgical evacuation is considered.

Ventricular Catheter Infections

A high risk of meningitis is associated with placement of a ventricular catheter. The most common organism is Staphylococcus epidermidis (coagulase-negative). Most physicians would start prophylactic antibiotics using cefazolin (1 gm every 8 hours) or oxacillin (2 gm every 6 hours), treating as long as the ventricular catheter is in place. Meningitis presents as fever and change in the level of consciousness. Diagnosis can be made by CSF aspirated through the ventricular catheter. Treatment is with intravenous vancomycin (1 gm every 12 hours) or oxacillin (2 gm every 4 hours).

4

Adult Medical Intensive Care

Peter Rock, James Shear

INITIAL ASSESSMENT

Critically ill patients have a failure of one or more organ systems that puts their lives in jeopardy within a short period without intervention. The organ failure may be acute or acute superimposed upon chronic disease and can have a negative impact on other organ systems. Most commonly, the initial recognition of critical illness involves a failure of the cardiovascular or pulmonary system, although any organ failure may result in a patient's admission to an ICU. Signs and symptoms of organ failure must be recognized, intervention undertaken, and a cause sought to treat the patient and return them to baseline status. When a patient arrives in the ICU, priorities must be established, a focused resuscitation performed, and further patient information acquired. Time must not be wasted searching for information before resuscitative efforts; these must proceed simultaneously. The goal is to determine the cause of the illness to determine the treatment of the critical condition.

Initial assessment and evaluation begins with resuscitation and stabilization. The basic ABCs of life support, airway, breathing, and circulation, are addressed first. Assessment is made of each and intervention undertaken as needed. After stabilization, a more thorough history is acquired, a physical examination is performed, and data is obtained, including blood chemistries, hematologic status, various imaging studies, and cardiac evaluation with an ECG or echocardiogram as indicated.

Assessing a patient's mental status is a high priority. Many critically ill patients have somnolence and obtundation or may present in a comatose state. For these patients, resuscitation and stabilization takes precedence. For a more stable patient who presents with a normal mental state, a more conservative approach may be taken, starting with gathering diagnostic information for a database for the patient's further treatment.

The care of critically ill patients is always a team approach. Multiple tasks must be undertaken simultaneously with one member acting as a leader, orchestrating and prioritizing the tasks. While the patient's mental status is being assessed, other members of the critical care team obtain vital signs to determine the patient's homeostatic impairment. Life support, such as CPR, is performed as needed, regardless of the underlying cause. The initial mental status assessment determines the need for and type of resuscitation, which should be carried out in a logical and sequential manner.

RESUSCITATION

Resuscitation begins with the familiar "ABCs," regardless of the cause or need for life support. Standard protocols have been developed and are part of Basic Life Support (BLS) and Advanced Cardiac Life Support (ACLS) courses.

Airway

Patients should be assessed for airway patency and for their ability to "protect" the airway. An obstructed airway will not allow air to pass and, therefore, must be relieved. Blood or secretions may be removed by suctioning. Alteration in the position of the airway, using the jaw-thrust and head-tilt maneuver, can relieve obstruction caused by the tongue falling back in the pharynx in the obtunded patient. This may be all that is necessary to relieve an obstruction to airflow in an otherwise spontaneously breathing patient. Adjuncts, such as an oral or nasal airway, may help relieve airway obstruction. If the previous efforts are unsuccessful, an artificial airway may be necessary with placement of an endotracheal tube (ETT) or, surgically, with a cricothyrotomy or tracheotomy.

Placement of an endotracheal tube by direct laryngoscopy is the first line of treatment for a patient in whom other measures to ensure a patent airway are unsuccessful. Patients who are breathing spontaneously through an unobstructed airway, but are obtunded or comatose and at risk for aspiration because of loss of airway reflexes, should also be considered candidates for endotracheal tube placement. Evaluating the patient for ease or difficulty of placement requires examination of the patient's mouth and neck. Proper positioning of the patient for successful placement of the endotracheal tube by direct laryngoscopy requires a mouth opening of at least 5 cm ("three-finger breaths") and the ability to extend the neck approximately 30°. Intubation should be carried out by an individual skilled in the procedure. If the patient's anatomy does not permit intubation by direct laryngoscopy, other methods for securing the airway should be considered, including fiberoptic laryngoscopy, cricotyrotomy, or tracheotomy.

Laryngoscopy and intubation are potentially noxious procedures that can produce sympathetic stimulation. Increases in heart rate, blood pressure, and intracranial pressure may cause deleterious effects in patients with coronary artery or cerebrovascular disease. Myocardial ischemia or failure may develop, as well as cerebral hemorrhage. In addition, any preexisting elevation in intracranial pressure may be exacerbated during laryngoscope and intubation resulting in brainstem herniation. The sympathetic responses can be attenuated by analgesics, sedatives, hypnotics, topical anesthetics, antihypertensives, or β-blockers, using careful titration to maintain homeostasis. Neuromuscular blockers (muscle relaxants) may be necessary for intubation in a patient to attain proper positioning and mouth opening, and to relax the vocal cords.

Patients who require emergent intubation always are considered to have "full stomachs" and are at increased risk for regurgitation and aspiration that may result in a severe pneumonitis; therefore, precautions must be taken to prevent this. Cricoid pressure is applied during laryngoscopy and intubation. Pressure is placed on the cricoid ring, pressing it against the esophagus and preventing stomach contents from reaching the posterior pharynx. Once intubation is completed, confirmation of proper tube placement is necessary. Unrecognized esophageal intubation may be fatal if not detected in a timely manner. Confirmation of proper placement of the endotracheal tube requires the presence of bilateral breath sounds, bilateral chest expansion, condensation ("misting") in the endotracheal tube, a lack of sounds over the stomach and, most importantly, the presence of carbon dioxide in exhaled gas measured by a capnometer.

Breathing

If airway patency has been assured, then breathing, the "B" in "ABC," is evaluated. If patency is questionable, the preceding procedures should be instituted. Breathing is evaluated by checking for visible respiratory efforts, listening for breath sounds, and gauging the adequacy of respiratory efforts and gas exchange. Skin color is an important indication of adequate oxygenation. Cyanosis, detected most easily in the nailbeds, reveals a profound decrease in hemoglobin saturation. Severe anemia may mask cyanosis, because approximately 5 g/dL of hemoglobin are necessary to produce this physical finding.

Respiratory rate is an important parameter to evaluate. Too slow a rate (less than 6) may indicate respiratory depression from a number of different causes and may lead to hypoventilation, hypercarbia, and hypoxemia. Hyperventilation (more than 30) may be caused by inadequate oxygenation, increased oxygen demand, or increased dead space and may lead to respiratory fatigue and failure. If respiratory efforts are not adequate, then ventilation must be assisted or controlled with a mask-bag device or an endotracheal tube and a self-inflating bag valve unit.

The patient's airway and chest should be examined to determine treatable causes for impaired ventilation, oxygenation, or both. Common causes include airway obstruction, pneumothorax, pneumonia, congestive heart failure, or severe anemia. Systemic conditions, such as sepsis, also can result in respiratory compromise. Adequate resuscitation requires discovering treatable causes and treating them effectively. Quantitative analysis of oxygenation and ventilation should be obtained as soon as possible using an arterial blood gas sample. Continuous monitoring with a pulse oximeter and a capnograph (if the patient is intubated and on mechanical ventilatory support) enables continuous assessment of oxygenation and ventilation and patient responses to changes in management. Observation and mechanical ventilation, if necessary, should be continued and periodic reassessments should be made to determine the adequacy of gas exchange.

Circulation

Cardiopulmonary Resuscitation

When a patent airway and breathing are assured either by natural or artificial means, the adequacy of circulation and perfusion must be addressed. The ability of the lungs to oxygenate the blood takes precedence over the ability of the blood to perfuse the organs ("B" comes before "C"). Circulation without pulmonary oxygenation is futile. Vital signs, evaluated during the initial assessment, determine whether adequate circulation is present. If not, as evidenced by the confirmed lack of pulse, CPR must be instituted promptly, because the timeliness of CPR is related to its efficacy and the patient's survival. If circulation is present, then the adequacy of perfusion needs to be assessed by palpating pulses and measuring blood pressure.

The goal is to assure adequate perfusion. CPR may be instituted even in the presence of a weak arterial pulse and a low blood pressure, if the perfusion is inadequate to sustain vital organs. This is determined by examination of the patient's mental status, skin color, temperature (especially of the extremities), and urine output. Venous access should be secured as rapidly as possible, because intravenous access is important for the administration of fluids and the pharmacologic treatment of cardiopulmonary arrest. Large bore peripheral venous lines may be sufficient unless vasoactive drugs are necessary. For this, a central line should be placed that also will allow measurement of central venous pressures and the placement of a pulmonary artery catheter, if necessary. The central line may be placed in the internal jugular, subclavian, or femoral veins as the need and opportunity exists. Initial resuscitation of most patients can be performed with peripheral intravenous access and should not be delayed to start a central venous catheter.

ASSESSMENT OF HYPOTENSION

The differential diagnosis of hypotension can be divided into three categories. In the ICU setting, *hypovolemia* most commonly results from hemorrhage, either from upper or lower GI sources. Hypovolemia also may result from insensible losses or unreplaced urinary losses. Patients who are hypovolemic will manifest decreased urine output (oliguria), flat neck veins, poor skin turgor, and orthostatic vital signs. Central venous pressure may be used to confirm the diagnosis. A low hematocrit with hypotension suggests acute blood loss. However, a decrease in hematocrit may not occur immediately after an acute loss of blood. The possibility of a GI hemorrhage should investigated by looking for blood in the stomach (NG tube aspirate) or in the stool.

Impaired cardiac function also may cause hypotension. Thus, an acute myocardial infarction or ongoing myocardial ischemia may present with decreased blood pressure. The typical symptoms of crushing chest pain and evidence of infarction or ischemia can establish the diagnosis. Drugs (β-blockers) and severe hypoxemia also may result in decreased cardiac function.

Decreased systemic vascular resistance (SVR) is the other category in the differential diagnosis of hypotension. So called "vasculogenic" hypotension is usually the result of bacterial infection and sepsis. Patients with sepsis and hypotension usually have relatively normal cardiac function. Intravascular volume is decreased relative to the increased capacity of the vascular bed, but is not the primary cause of lowered blood pressure. Blood pressure is related to cardiac output by resistance (Ohm's law, SVR = [MAP − CVP]/CO). At a given level of cardiac output, reductions in SVR decreases blood pressure. The diagnosis of sepsis and decreased SVR is suggested by a compatible clinical site of infection (e.g., pneumonia, peritonitis) and no obvious source of hemorrhage. Sepsis and decreased SVR may be confirmed by measuring SVR with a pulmonary artery catheter. Another cause of decreased SVR is spinal shock, seen in patients with high spinal cord injuries that result in loss of vascular tone.

Other causes of hypotension include pulmonary embolus (obstructing outflow from RV), pericardial effusion or tamponade, and tension pneumothorax. Most causes of hypotension can be incorporated into the three preceding diagnostic frameworks listed.

Fluid Resuscitation

Treatment with intravenous fluids is an effective intervention in the initial management of critically ill patients and the response to such treatment provides rapid diagnostic information. In patients with no or inadequate perfusion, the aggressive administration of intravenous fluids may increase cardiac output and perfusion of vital organs with a reversal of hypotension. Improved circulation enhances oxygen delivery to the tissues. A decrease in tissue hypoxia should have a salutary effect on organ failure and lead to improvement. Although the thesis that treatments aimed at increasing oxygen delivery (above normal) will improve patient outcome is theoretically attractive, it has not been confirmed experimentally.

Fluids may be necessary for a number of reasons. An inadequate amount of fluid may be in the vascular compartments, such as occurs with hemorrhage or burns. The amount of fluid in the body may be adequate, but its location may make it unavailable to the vascular space, such as occurs with "third spacing" of fluids in trauma or after surgery. The ability of the heart to pump blood to vital organs, including itself, may be impaired, as seen in sepsis (usually modest effect), myocardial infarction, or other conditions that depress cardiac function. Patients with impaired heart function require increased "filling" pressures, which is achieved by fluid administration.

Fluid administration is necessary to improve circulation and, therefore, is important to oxygen delivery because it improves cardiac output. Fluid challenges are accomplished by administering boluses of intravenous fluids rapidly, e.g., 250 mL over 10 to 15 minutes. The effects of such interventions are an increase in blood pressure, a decrease in heart rate, or an increase in urine output; any or all of these would indicate a positive response to the fluid challenge. Many critically ill patients will require large amounts of fluid to restore circulatory equilibrium.

The use of a central line or pulmonary artery catheter can help in assessing the effects of fluid administration, guiding further therapy, and determining the filling pressure at which circulation is enhanced and oxygen delivery is improved. These monitors also can prevent excessive intravascular pressures that can lead to increased pulmonary hydrostatic pressure and consequent pulmonary congestion.

The choice of fluid to administer depends on the clinical circumstances. A patient who has lost a significant amount of blood will require packed red blood cells. Patients with losses to the extravascular space can be replenished with either crystalloid or colloid. The two most common colloids used in volume expansion are 5% albumin and 6% hydroxyethyl starch. Colloidal fluids are able, because of their oncotic properties, to expand the intravascular volume to a greater extent, with less volume, than crystalloids. Crystalloid fluids move more rapidly from the vascular space into the interstitium than colloidal fluids; therefore, less remains in the intravascular space to be available for the circulation. Two or three times the amount of colloid is necessary if crystalloid is used to expand the intravascular space. However, the efficacy of crystalloid versus colloid, in terms of outcome, has not been established. Although concerns of colloids causing harm in acute lung injury have been refuted and colloids have been shown to cause less interstitial edema than crystalloids, crystalloids are nevertheless efficacious and safe and, therefore, the additional cost of colloids may not be justified.

Once a critically ill patient has been resuscitated adequately and stabilized, efforts can be directed at determining the underlying causes of their illness and developing a database for further diagnosis, treatment, and prognosis.

RESPIRATORY FAILURE

The two major categories of respiratory insufficiency are oxygenation impairment and ventilatory failure. Patients who have primary difficulty with oxygenation may still be able to ventilate normally (i.e., excrete CO_2). The acute respiratory distress syndrome (ARDS) is most often seen with other disease states such as sepsis, trauma, aspiration, severe pneumonia, or shock from other causes. ARDS is characterized by oxygenation failure with refractory hypoxemia, diffuse lung injury with diffuse pulmonary infiltrates on chest radiograph, and decreased lung compliance. This acute lung injury is manifest as pulmonary edema from increased permeability of the pulmonary endothelium. Because there is no specific treatment for ARDS, supportive therapy is used. Mechanical ventilation may exacerbate the lung injury associated with ARDS by stretching the lung or other forms of barotrauma. Thus, mechanical ventilation may be adjusted to minimize lung inflation and deflation.

The degree of oxygenation impairment can be characterized by the alveolar-arterial oxygen tension gradient (A-a Do_2). This reflects the ability of the pulmonary alveoli to oxygenate the blood that passes through them. The normal difference is ~ 10 mm Hg and increases slightly with age. An increased gradient represents impaired gas exchange.

Pulmonary embolus can cause severe hypoxemia from changes in ventilation-perfusion relationships caused by vasoactive substances from the embolus. Other causes of hypoxemia are shunts (e.g., Ventricular Septal Defects [VSD]) or impaired diffusion in patients with advanced forms of interstitial lung disease.

Ventilatory failure is characterized by difficulty in eliminating CO_2. Common ICU conditions in which this is observed are asthma and chronic obstructive pulmonary disease (COPD) both of which obstruct expiratory airflow. With asthma, the obstruction is a reversible defect treatable with bronchodilators and anti-inflammatory agents (corticosteroids). COPD is a more fixed disorder related to the destruction of lung parenchyma. Neuromuscular diseases weaken the respiratory muscles causing an inability to eliminate CO_2 . Alterations in level of consciousness produced by cerebral vascular accidents (CVAs) or intoxication may also cause ventilatory failure by interfering with the drive to ventilate.

MECHANICAL VENTILATION

The ability to insert an artificial airway and maintain the patient on mechanical ventilation is one of the major advances in modern critical-care medicine. The inspired concentration of oxygen, FiO_2, should be established. In a critically ill individual in whom the oxygenation status is uncertain the patient can breathe 100% oxygen until arterial blood gases or other measures of arterial oxygen saturation can be used to guide further changes in FiO_2 .

The amount of each breath and tidal volume also is set. Patients receive a tidal volume of 10 to 12 mL/kg of body weight. Although this is larger than the size of a breath of a normal resting individual, such tidal volumes are necessary to overcome the compliance of the ventilator circuit and to insure adequate ventilation. Individuals who are either small or morbidly obese may require some deviation from these guidelines. Tidal volume should be based on ideal body weight.

Mechanical ventilators have several "modes" of ventilation. *Assist control* can be used when the patient is making no spontaneous respiratory efforts. In this mode, the patient receives a preset number of mechanical breaths at a preset tidal volume. If the patient attempts to initiate additional breaths, the ventilator will assist the patient giving a full "machine" breath. The patient does not have to expend much energy because all patient breaths in their entirety are performed by the ventilator whether initiated spontaneously or by machine.

Synchronized intermittent mandatory ventilation (SIMV) will deliver a preset number of breaths to the patient as well. In this mode of ventilation, the machine will attempt to "time" machine breaths with patient attempts at spontaneous breaths, thus reducing the potential for barotrauma and, theoretically, making the patient more comfortable. Between the machine-mandated breaths, the patient may breathe spontaneously, therefore, the work of breathing may be high depending on the number of spontaneous breaths the patient attempts, the resistance associated with the ventilator circuit, the resistance of the patient airways, and respiratory system compliance. Spontaneous breaths in this mode of ventilation are not assisted by the ventilator.

Most modern ventilators are volume-cycled ventilators in that a "machine" breath is terminated (regardless of mode) after a preset volume of gas is delivered. *Pressure-support* ventilation often is used to assist patients and to facilitate weaning from mechanical ventilation. Pressure-support ventilation initially delivers a high flow rate of gas so that a preset level of airway pressure is achieved. As the lungs fill, less flow is needed to maintain the level of airway pressure. Eventually, airflow decreases to a predetermined level, and the breath is terminated (a form of flow "cycling").

Mechanical ventilators are adjusted so that time required for inspiration is less than that required for exhalation. A normal I:E ratio is approximately 1:2 or 1:2.5. Exhalation is passive and cannot be speeded up. Therefore, changes in the I:E ratio are achieved by adjusting the rate of inspiratory gas flow. *Inverse ratio ventilation (IRV)* is used in patients with severe lung disease and difficulties in oxygenation. This method of ventilation results in larger lung volumes and higher levels of mean intrathoracic pressure, and because it is uncomfortable for patients, it usually is administered in a sedated and paralyzed patient.

The number of breaths is set in either mode, usually starting at a rate of 12/minute. Depending on the tidal volume that has been selected and the patients underlying CO_2 production, the rate is then adjusted based on arterial blood gas analysis.

Positive end-expiratory pressure (PEEP), which is set in cm H_2O, can also be used in settings of oxygenation difficulty. Usually, PEEP is selected and arterial blood gases are measured after a period sufficient to establish relative constancy in pO_2 (in 20 minutes). If the pO_2 is not adequate, the PEEP is increased and ABCs are remeasured. PEEP, by holding alveoli and airways open, increases lung compliance. Thus, PEEP may be adjusted to optimize respiratory system compliance.

Mechanical ventilation may be associated with complications, such as the potential for barotrauma. Thus, patients on mechanical ventilation may suffer pneumothorax, often of a tension-type. Sudden hemodynamic compromise of a patient on mechanical ventilation should suggest pneumothorax. Rapid diagnosis (auscultation, CXR) and treatment (chest tube) are essential. Barotrauma also may take the form of subcutaneous emphysema that although present on CXR and on physical examination, frequently does not require emergent treatment.

The other major complication associated with mechanical ventilation is infection. Ventilator-associated pneumonia (VAP) is now a recognized entity. The endotracheal tube bypasses normal host defenses and provides a portal of entry for pathogens. Aspiration of oral or gastric contents also may occur because the cuff around an endotracheal tube (ETT) does not entirely prevent material from entering the lungs. Thus, patients need to be assessed and monitored vigorously for the possibility of VAP.

Patients on mechanical ventilation may have increased airway resistance (bronchospasm). Bronchodilators may be used to decrease airway resistance and improve ventilation. In the absence of wheezing audible by auscultation, a difference of more than 10 cm H_2O between peak and plateau airway pressure at an inspiratory flow rate of 60 L/minute suggests possible bronchospasm. Commonly used bronchodilators are nebulized into the airway. Commonly, β_2 selective agents are administered, although anticholinergic agents may be used in certain settings (COPD). Bronchodilators may cause tachycardia and increase the tenacity of airway secretions.

SEPSIS SYNDROME

Although confusion surrounds the terminology used in describing patients with sepsis, bacteremia, septic shock, endotoxemia, etc., it is important to develop definitions that allow clinical identification to expedite treatment and allow for ongoing research into the causes, prevention, and treatment of Sepsis Syndrome. A systemic inflammatory response to many different clinical insults, Sepsis Syndrome is also known as Systemic Inflammatory Response Syndrome (SIRS). Patients with Sepsis Syndrome may or may not have bacteremia and may present with a large variety of clinical conditions, including hyper or hypothermia, tachycardia, increased or decreased cardiac output, tachypnea, hypoxemia, mental status changes, renal insufficiency, leukocytosis, thrombocytopenia, coagulopathy, hyperglycemia, or acidosis. Patients may present with one or many of these conditions and need to be observed closely and treated aggressively if Sepsis Syndrome is suspected.

Patients with Sepsis Syndrome may present awake and alert and hemodynamically stable or obtunded and in shock. Those who are unstable require aggressive resuscitation and support. History is extremely important in determining if Sepsis Syndrome is present and the physical examination is important in determining the severity of the condition and the appropriate treatment. Early treatment with antibiotics is essential. Because cultures are usually not available for 1 to 2 days, empiric treatment must be carried out based on the most likely organisms to be cultured. This is based on the history and physical examination, the patient's presentation, gram stain results, and specific susceptibilities within a given hospital, especially for patients hospitalized prior to developing Sepsis Syndrome. Support within an ICU is essential with close monitoring and vigorous support in the form of mechanical ventilation, fluid resuscitation, hemodynamic monitoring, and pharmacologic treatment of cardiovascular compromise. In addition, nutritional support, especially in the form of enteral feeding, is an increasingly important factor in the prognosis of patients with Sepsis Syndrome. Sepsis remains a leading cause for ICU admissions and deaths in ICUs.

ASSESSMENT OF HEMODYNAMIC VARIABLES

Critically ill patients with abnormalities of blood pressure and/or cardiac function may require invasive assessment of these parameters. An intra-arterial catheter can be used to measure blood pressure continuously and accurately, although noninvasive techniques may be used unless severe hypotension is present. Arterial catheters have the advantage of a continuous display and permit arterial blood sampling.

A pulmonary artery catheter is a balloon-tipped catheter with several internal lumen. One lumen terminates at the distal end of the device (distal or PA), and when properly positioned, the device can be used to measure pulmonary artery pressure. Another lumen terminates approximately 20 cm from the tip, and when the catheter is in the correct position, it can measure right atrial pressure (proximal or RA). A thermistor is also at the end of the catheter. The balloon has two primary purposes. The first is to position the catheter in the pulmonary artery (PA). The catheter is introduced in the central circulation via a vein leading to the central circulation (e.g., internal jugular, subclavian, or femoral vein). Then, the balloon is inflated. It acts as "sail" and is carried by the flow of blood through the right-sided heart chambers and into the pulmonary artery.

After correct positioning in the PA, inflation of the balloon results in distal migration of the catheter until it obstructs a small branch of the PA ("wedges"). This results in no flow of blood through this branch of the PA, capillaries, and small pulmonary veins served by this branch of the PA. A static column of blood is created from pulmonary veins to the distal lumen of the catheter. The PA lumen thus "senses" pulmonary vein pressure. Because this portion of the pulmonary circulation has a low resistance, pulmonary venous pressure is close to left atrial pressure, which is close to left ventricular end-diastolic pressure under conditions of normal valvular function. Right atrial and pulmonary capillary wedge (PCW) pressures are referred to as "filling pressures" because they reflect the filling or loading conditions of the right and left atrium respectively.

Cardiac output can be measured using the PA catheter. An indicator dilution technique is employed using a cold injection through the proximal lumen. The "cold" is the indicator and is diluted by the cardiac output. The thermistor at the tip of the catheter detects temperature changes. A specialized computer then determines the cardiac output based on the area under the temperature–time curve.

Complications of PA catheters are related to the insertion and passage of the device. Gaining access to the central circulation can be associated with arterial puncture (carotid or subclavian) or pneumothorax. As the catheter is "floated" into position, arrhythmia's, especially ventricular tachycardia, or right bundle branch block may be observed. Long-term use of the device may be associated with catheter-related infection, sepsis, and thrombosis.

The PA catheter is most valuable in helping determine the cause of hypotension and can help the clinician determine whether hypovolemia, myocardial dysfunction, or vasculogenic hypotension is present. Low RA and PCW pressures and increased SVR suggest hypovolemia. An elevated PCW associated with a decreased cardiac output suggests myocardial dysfunction. Low filling pressures and normal or low SVR suggests sepsis.

PA catheters are not designed to supplant clinical acumen but rather to supplement it. The ability of clinicians to assess filling pressures and cardiac output without the aid of supplemental devices is poor, especially in critically ill patients. However, there is no evidence that PA catheters have actually reduced mortality in critically ill patients, and there is some evidence that they may worsen outcome. Thus, the risks and benefits of PA catheters must be assessed carefully whenever considering their use.

VASOACTIVE DRUGS

Patients in the ICU often require cardiovascular system support to maintain adequate perfusion of vital organs. When fluid support alone is not successful in maintaining an adequate cardiac output and blood pressure, vasoactive agents may be necessary. Drugs that increase vasomotor tone or SVR are used frequently. Dopamine is a commonly used first-line agent for treating hypotension and is a catecholamine, which at low doses < μg/kg per minute) produces renal artery vasodilation, at intermediate doses (3 to 10 μg/kg per minute) produces β-agonist activity, and at high doses (> 10 μg/kg per minute) stimulates α-receptors. Dopamine raises SVR and cardiac output but may cause tachycardia or dysrhythmias. Other vasoactive agents include phenylephrine, which is a pure α-agonist and increases SVR without increasing heart rate; rather, a reflex bradycardia may develop. Norepinephrine is a potent α vasoconstrictor that is often used at low doses with dopamine to attempt to ameliorate the severe vasoconstriction of the renal arteries caused by norepinephrine.

Epinephrine, an α- and β-agonist, is used for hypotension when cardiac causes are suspected. When hypotension from cardiac causes and decreased perfusion are confirmed, by pulmonary artery catheter monitoring, inotropic agents are used to boost the contractility of the heart. A commonly used agent is dobutamine that mainly stimulates β-receptors, causing mild afterload reduction allowing for greater cardiac output. Amrinone, a phosphodiesterase inhibitor, and digoxin also increase cardiac output. Vasodilating agents, such as nitroprusside, nitroglycerine, or angiotensin-converting enzyme (ACE) inhibitors, are used to decrease blood pressure in significantly hypertensive patients, produce afterload reduction in patients with congestive heart failure, or in the case of nitroglycerin, improve blood flow to the coronary arteries.

ASSESSMENT OF ORGAN FUNCTION

The kidneys, liver, and CNS may be profoundly affected by changes in cardiac output and/or hypotension. In turn, diseases of any of these three critical organs may result in admission to a critical care unit. Renal function may be readily assessed using a few available indices. Urinary output, when preserved (and without "stimulation" by diuretics), demonstrates the adequacy of renal perfusion and thus the adequacy of intravascular volume. Decreased urine output thus suggests decreased renal perfusion as a result of either hypovolemia or decreased cardiac output. Increases in blood urea nitrogen (BUN) out of proportion to creatinine suggest hypovolemia (BUN:Creatinine > 20). Elevations of both BUN and creatinine maintaining a 10:1 ratio suggest primary renal dysfunction. Hyperkalemia may be seen in renal dysfunction from any cause and merits close observation and treatment if necessary.

Hepatic function can be assessed by measuring several blood chemicals. The coagulation factors, synthesized primarily by the liver, are sensitive indicators of hepatic synthetic function abnormalities. The presence of a coagulopathy should alert the clinician to the possibility of hepatic dysfunction. Reductions in albumin in the absence of obvious malnutrition and/or the nephrotic syndrome also indicate impaired hepatic synthetic ability. An increase in hepatic cell enzymes, such as AST and ALT, indicate liver injury from a variety of causes including decreased perfusion. Bilirubin is increased in liver dysfunction because the ability of the liver to clear bile pigments is impaired. Two liver-related compounds, ammonia and lactate, are factors in this condition. Ammonia levels increase in patients with severe liver dysfunction. This increase not only helps diagnose liver failure, but also may explain changes in mental state such as obtundation in a critically ill patient. Lactate, a product of anaerobic metabolism, is cleared by the liver. Patients with liver disease may not metabolize this compound normally and may demonstrate elevated levels of lactate exacerbating an underlying metabolic acidosis.

COMA

Patients may present to the ICU in a coma (see Chapter 3). The term coma represents a significantly depressed level of consciousness with a total absence of awareness of surroundings. The patient is unresponsive to external stimulation, even pain. Coma may result from significant depression or injury to the bilateral cortical area or the brainstem. Structural changes, usually the result of space-occupying lesions, may also cause a coma. The structural changes may include intracranial hemorrhage, subdural hematoma, neoplasm, abscess, infarction, or swelling from other causes. Focal signs may be present in patients with coma from a structural cause. Nonstructural causes include infectious, toxic, and metabolic etiologies.

Infections causing meningitis may be bacterial or viral and can lead to coma, usually without lateralizing signs. Toxic causes include overdoses with drugs such as opioids, barbiturates, benzodiazepines, salicylates, acetaminophen, or poisons. Metabolic causes of coma include hypoglycemia, severe hyperglycemia, renal failure with uremia, hepatic failure, and anoxic brain injury.

Patients presenting with coma in the ICU are managed with aggressive support. The "ABCs" are followed and patients are treated to maintain hemodynamic stability as necessary. Patients who are comatose require endotracheal intubation for airway protection to prevent aspiration pneumonitis. History obtained from family or friends and physical examination is important to determine the cause of the comatose state. Laboratory studies are used as well as imaging techniques to determine the cause and the proper therapy. A lumbar puncture, after CNS space-occupying lesions are excluded, may reveal meningitis.

ENDOCRINE/METABOLIC

Diabetic Ketoacidosis (DKA) generally occurs in patients with insulin dependent (type 1) diabetes. The lack of insulin coupled with other etiologic disorders, such as infection, may result in impairment of glucose use; altered metabolism resulting in ketogenesis; increased anion gap acidosis; and hyperglycemia resulting in glucosuria causing an osmotic diuresis leading to severe dehydration, hypokalemia, and hypertonicity. Patients may present with weakness, mental status changes, polyuria, polydipsia, nausea and vomiting, tachypnea, tachycardia, and signs of severe dehydration. Patients with DKA typically have as much as a 5-L fluid deficit, while at the same time produce copious amounts of urine. Laboratory findings include an increased glucose (400 to 1000 mg/dL), glucosuria, hypokalemia (total body depletion that may initially appear normal), hypophosphatemia, metabolic alkalosis with an increased anion gap, ketonemia, and hyponatremia based upon the level of glucose. Treatment requires supplementing insulin, usually in the form of a continuous infusion, replenishing fluids with aggressive replacement, potassium replacement, and phosphate repletion. A search for triggering causes should be undertaken, which may include infection, often pulmonary, cardiac disease, such as myocardial infarction, or trauma. Often, no precipitating cause can be found.

GASTROINTESTINAL CONDITIONS

Gastrointestinal bleeding is a common cause of admission to an ICU. Upper GI (UGI) bleeding is caused by a number of conditions, including peptic ulcer disease, esophageal varices, gastric erosions and Mallory-Weiss tears. Peptic ulcers are a common cause and account for about one-half of all UGI bleeding. Treatment varies from endoscopic injection or cauterization, which is usually successful when a bleeding vessel is found, to surgical intervention when unsuccessful, or for continued hemorrhage. Esophageal varices from portal hypertension may present as UGI bleeding. Diagnosis by endoscopy allows for treatment with sclerotherapy. If unsuccessful, vasopressin may be administered to attempt to stop bleeding from varices. Balloon tamponade with one of a number of devices may help stop bleeding until specific treatment is available. Surgical procedures may be necessary either emergently or electively for patients with multiple episodes. Since these patients typically have liver disease a coagulopathy may exist and should be corrected. Gastric erosions are common in patients with critical illness and UGI bleeding is a common sequelae. Treatment of the underlying critical illness is the key to prevention; however, H_2-receptor antagonists generally are used prophylactically to decrease acid production. Mallory-Weiss tears occur after significant vomiting often associated with alcohol abuse. This usually requires only supportive treatment such as fluids; however, it may require endoscopic or surgical treatment.

Lower GI bleeding is usually related to polyps, diverticular disease, cancer or AVMs. Diagnosis may be made by colonoscopy, although angiography or radionuclide studies may be necessary. Bleeding may be halted endoscopically with cautery or laser therapy. Polypectomy is also achieved endoscopically. Intra-arterial administration of vasopressin may be an option but has significant limitations. Surgery is necessary if bleeding continues and may be done emergently or electively if bleeding is slow and the patient is stable.

Pancreatitis may be caused by a number of conditions, including alcoholism, infection, or drugs, or it may be idiopathic.

Patients may require ICU admission for hemodynamic instability, generally because of volume depletion secondary to fluid shifts. Treatment is generally supportive and the clinical course may include severe instability requiring vasoactive treatment and mechanical ventilatory support. Severe pancreatitis with neurosis may require surgical debridement.

Acute Renal Failure

Acute renal failure (ARF) occurs commonly in patients critically ill from a variety of causes (approximately 20% incidence in ICU population). The presence of renal failure combined with respiratory failure is associated with high mortality rates. The function of the kidney can be performed by mechanical means (dialysis) and, to a certain extent, physiologic compensation occurs when there is renal insufficiency. Thus, kidney failure usually is not immediately lethal. However, renal failure is often an ominous development in patients who are ill from other causes.

Renal function can be assessed by measuring urine output (a crude measure of renal perfusion) and blood concentrations of urea nitrogen (BUN) and creatinine. Patients that are producing adequate amounts of urine (> 0.5 mL/kg per hour) probably have adequate renal perfusion, although oliguria may occur from causes other than inadequate renal perfusion. When the kidneys acutely fail, each day, BUN increases ~ 10 mg/dL, and creatinine increases to ~ 1 mg/dL. The rate of increase of these compounds is also a function of the patient's catabolic and nutritional states. Importantly, potassium will increase and bicarbonate will decrease in patients with acute renal failure.

Stabilization in previously increasing BUN and creatinine levels reflect a new equilibrium between the production and elimination of each, implying stabilization in the level of renal perfusion and glomerular perfusion rates at new, lower than normal levels. Normally BUN:Creatinine is 10. Increases suggest prerenal causes of deterioration in renal function (decreased renal perfusion secondary to inadequate intravascular volume), whereas a ratio of 10 in the presence of adequate intravascular volume suggests renal causes. The ability of the kidneys to concentrate urine also is impaired in the presence of ARF and whereas the normal kidney can reduce urinary sodium to less than 20 mEq/L, the failing kidney will produce urine with much higher levels of urinary sodium.

Causes of ARF can be divided into prerenal, renal, and postrenal conditions. Prerenal causes of ARF usually are related to factors that decrease renal perfusion, which include decreases in blood pressure, decreased cardiac output, and vascular conditions such as an aortic aneurysm. Renal causes of ARF include glomerulonephritis from any cause, interstitial nephritis seen with use of certain drugs, and ATN secondary to drugs. Nephrotoxic drugs, such as aminoglycosides, are a common cause of ARF. Other agents that may precipitate ARF include NSAIDs, radiographic contrast agents, ACE inhibitors, and myoglobin and hemoglobin if they are released into the bloodstream from cellular breakdown. Postrenal causes of ARF include ureteral obstruction from calculi or retroperitoneal masses.

Patients with ARF require careful attention to their fluid and electrolyte status to ensure that life-threatening hyperkalemia does not occur and to prevent fluid overload. Low-dose dopamine (< 5 μg/kg per minute) may be used to improve renal perfusion. Reduced potassium intake and potassium-binding resins administered via the GI tract may help control hyperkalemia. Dialysis may be required to remove excess fluid, control electrolyte concentrations and remove products of metabolism. Ultrafiltration is a technique best suited for removal of intravascular volume. Hemodialysis is used when large amounts of toxins and fluid have to be removed or when rapid correction of abnormal chemistries is required.

Patients with ARF are at increased risk for the development of infection. In addition, acute and potentially life-threatening bleeding may occur in patients with ARF as a result of impaired platelet function from this condition.

5

Surgical Intensive Care

Clifford S. Deutschman

Management of patients in the surgical intensive care unit (SICU) is based on the maintenance of an airway, adequate ventilation, and preservation of cardiovascular parameters as discussed throughout this book. In addition, other issues are of particular concern in the SICU. Because surgery substantially alters physiology and metabolism, pattern recognition is especially important. In this chapter, we will outline the characteristic response that follows tissue trauma, either after injury (unanesthetized) or elective surgery (anesthetized). We will then discuss the implications of this response regarding management, the significance of common deviations from the expected response, and the impact of common preexisting diseases. This background provides a useful context upon which to acquire experience in the management of critically ill surgical patients.

PERIOPERATIVE STRESS RESPONSE

Our understanding of the perioperative stress response comes from the landmark work of several groups of investigators. The initial description was published in 1932 by David Cuthbertson, who has since devoted a lifetime of work to understanding perioperative physiology. Cuthbertson noted that body temperature in patients with long bone fractures followed a characteristic trajectory. In the first 24 hours after injury, temperature declined. It returned to baseline and then rose, reaching a peak on about the third postinjury day. In the absence of complications, temperature returned to baseline by postinjury day 7. Cuthbertson reasoned that temperature reflected metabolic rate. Subsequent work has demonstrated that this characteristic trajectory is reflected in many physiologic and metabolic parameters (Fig 5.1) . Cuthbertson dubbed the initial period of decreased metabolism the "Ebb" phase, reflecting the decrease in metabolism. Subsequently, he discovered change in the distribution of peripheral blood flow, naming this second phase the "Flow" phase.

Teleologically, the response is appropriate and adaptive. The initial phase that we now term shock is designed to prevent death. This requires intense support of the heart and central nervous system. Thus, blood flow to these most vital organs is preserved at the expense of delivery to all other organ systems. Such a situation obviously cannot persist for long, and if shock persists, death becomes inevitable. Therefore, endogenous mechanisms to prevent further volume loss (hemostasis) and expand the blood volume are activated. If substrate delivery to the heart and the brain become adequate, flow is sequentially restored to other vascular beds (kidneys, then liver and gut, then muscle, then skin). This, in turn, initiates the second stage of the response.

The driving force behind the second phase of the stress response, now referred to as the phase of hypermetabolism, is repair of damaged tissue. This is an energy-requiring process and primarily reflects the increased metabolic activity of white blood cells, which are recruited to injured areas. White cells are fueled almost exclusively by glucose. Thus, endogenous mechanisms that increase glucose availability and limit glucose use by tissues other than white cells are activated. Glycogen from muscle and liver is mobilized rapidly. Hepatic gluconeogenesis is stimulated and substrate for this process is provided by the breakdown of skeletal and visceral muscle to polypeptides and amino acids. These gluconeogenic precursors are delivered to the liver via enhanced blood flow. In effect, the body cannibalizes endogenous protein to support hypermetabolism. This

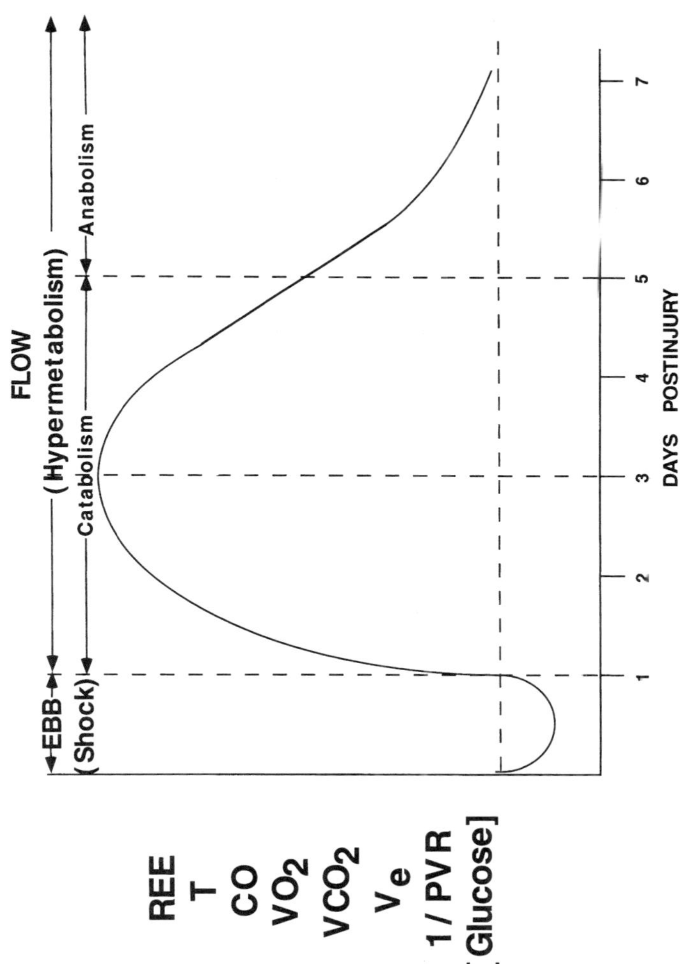

Figure 5.1. The stress response; pattern of changes in metabolic and physiologic parameters over time after surgery. *REE,* resting energy expenditure; *CO,* cardiac output; *VO_2,* oxygen consumption; *VCO_2,* carbon dioxide production; *Ve,* minute ventilation; *PVR,* peripheral vascular resistance.

process is exacerbated by the need for protein synthesis, both to increase the abundance of important enzymes and to provide substrate for proteins, such as collagen, needed to repair damaged tissue. Support of hepatic metabolism, as well as the demands of other tissues, is met by increased oxidation of fat and glutamine.

The delivery of glucose to activated white cells in the area of damage also requires an alteration of normal physiology. White cells—first neutrophils, then macrophages and, ultimately, lymphocytes—accumulate in injured tissue. These cells migrate to the site of injury via diapedesis and remove debris, contain infection, and lay down a matrix of collagen. Delivery of substrate to these cells requires the development of a concentration gradient. Further, both allowing diapedesis and supplying white cells with glucose require the recruitment of capillaries and the development of "capillary leak," that is, the loosening of junctions between endothelial cells. In major injuries or after extensive operations, recruitment and leak become generalized. There are two important ramifications of this generalized capillary recruitment and leak. First, lung water will increase and results in an alteration in oxygen exchange and the development of hypoxemia. Second, dependent lung regions will collapse; this is the "postoperative atelectasis," which is commonly believed to alter oxygenation. In fact, the increase in lung water in the alveolar septa causes both hypoxemia and atelectasis. The latter is simply an epiphenomenon.

More importantly, the generalized capillary recruitment and leak will result in a redistribution of body water (Fig. 5.2). The significance of this was first recognized by Moore, who examined the partition of water between the potassium-rich intracellular compartment and the sodium-rich extracellular space. This work led to the discovery that, for 3 to 4 days after injury, the extracellular space increases dramatically. Use of labeled red blood cells indicates at least a doubling of the intravascular compartment, whereas investigations with labeled Na^+ revealed an even more substantial expansion of the extracellular, extravascular (interstitial) space. While mechanisms to conserve sodium and water loss are activated, the bulk of the in-

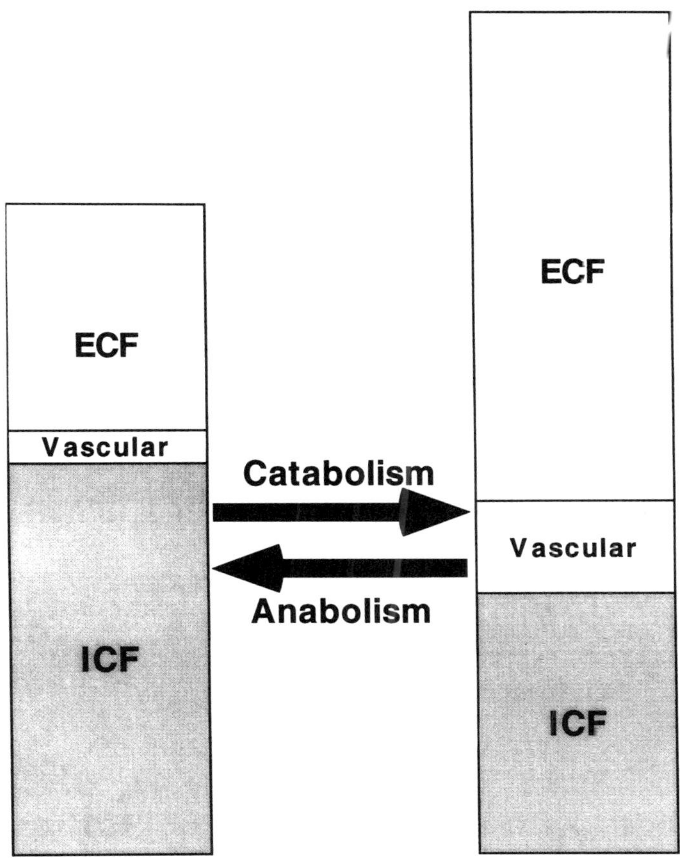

Figure 5.2. Changes in body water distribution after surgery. These changes reverse with the onset of the anabolic phase. *ECF*, extracellular fluid; *ICF*, intracellular fluid.

crease of fluid need is met by a decrease in intracellular water, evidenced by a loss of exchangeable K^+. Coupled with the loss of protein to supply the demands of hypermetabolism, this loss in intracellular water results in a substantial loss of body cell mass. Thus, Moore termed the initial period of hypermetabolism the "catabolic" phase. Moore also demonstrated that a transition occurred 3 to 4 days after the initial injury. At that time, the catabolic process began to reverse. Fluid moved from the extracellular to the intracellular compartment, excess fluid and sodium were excreted by the kidneys and electrolytes moved back into cells. This restoration of cell mass, which Moore called the "anabolic" phase, is clinically evidenced by diuresis and decreasing serum levels of the intracellular electrolytes K^+, Mg^{+2}, and PO_4^{-3}. Later work demonstrated that the catabolic process reversal reflects the neovascularization of damaged tissue, which takes about 4 days. Restoration of the vascular interface improves substrate delivery. Thus, the time course of the hypermetabolic is relatively fixed. The magnitude of the injury, however, determines the magnitude of the response.

The vasodilatation that results from the need to meet tissue demand alters cardiodynamics. Cardiac output increases both from stimulation of the contractile state and from loss of outflow impedance. The altered metabolic rate is reflected in increases in oxygen consumption and CO_2 production. Minute ventilation increases to facilitate CO_2 removal.

Understanding the stress response has important therapeutic implications. First, both trauma, when injury occurs in the absence of anesthesia, and elective, anesthetized surgery initiate the stress response by inducing shock. In trauma, this results from a reduction in cardiac output secondary to fluid loss, while in elective surgery, shock results from the use of a myocardial depressant and venodilating drugs; the net effect is the same, however. Shock is treatable with fluid administration. Thus, administration of volume to the patient will facilitate the transition from shock to hypermetabolism and can eliminate the Ebb phase effectively.

Unlike shock, the length of the hypermetabolic phase is determined by the need for neovascularization; therefore, the time course is fixed. However, studies attempting to decrease metabolic requirements with epidural anesthesia or α-adrenergic blockade have been unsuccessful. Epidural anesthesia for several days delays the onset of the hypermetabolic phase but does not alter its magnitude or duration. Use of clonidine does not alter nitrogen dynamics. However, pain can be managed well without adverse effect.

More importantly, hypermetabolism must be supported with appropriate fluid administration. This must be sufficient to keep up with losses into the "third space," that is, fluid that is directed to the extracellular space as a result of capillary leak. Anasarca may develop in postoperative patients, particularly those who are critically ill. However, this occurs at the expense of the intracellular and vascular compartments. Failure to administer fluids despite the appearance of "fluid overload" can result in shock, inadequate substrate delivery, and complications. Finally, administration of exogenous glucose cannot prevent cannibalization of endogenous nitrogen stores effectively. However, providing adequate protein will attenuate losses in severe cases. Thus, the sicker the patient, the more dependent on exogenous protein he or she becomes.

The transition from catabolism to anabolism is clinically evident and has therapeutic implications. As the capillary interface is restored, the demand for substrate delivery can be met directly, and the capillary leak resolves. The third-space fluid can be excreted. Thus, on the third or fourth postinjury/operative day, a brisk diuresis occurs accompanied by a decrease in serum electrolytes, which move back into cells. Consequently, serum levels of K^{+}, Mg^{+2} and PO_4^{-3} decrease and will need to be replenished. Now the discussion will focus on the abnormal.

Understanding the response to tissue injury allows prediction of the metabolic response and recognition that vasodilatation, increases in cardiac output, minute ventilation, hypoxemia, anasarca, and fever are normal. These changes are adaptive and need to be supported.

Deviations from the Response

Having established what is normal, the next step lies in recognizing patterns that are maladaptive. Deviations from the norm represent postoperative complications. The two most common deviations are a transition from hypermetabolism back to shock and a prolongation of the catabolic phase. Both may result from failure to give appropriate amounts of fluid. In that case, persistent hypoperfusion may produce organ dysfunction or simply precipitate shock. More commonly, a persistent inflammatory focus—an abscess, a gastrointestinal anastomotic leak, a large undrained hematoma, or an infectious focus such as a pneumonia or a contaminated intravenous catheter—results in a failure of transition from catabolism to anabolism. By definition, this constitutes the highly lethal systemic inflammatory response syndrome (SIRS)/multiple organ dysfunction syndrome (MODS), the most common causes of mortality and morbidity in critically ill surgical patients.

Persistent hypermetabolism often presents clinically with an inability to wean the patient from ventilatory support as a result of the high levels of minute ventilation required to excrete CO_2. Pulmonary compliance will remain abnormally low, and hypoxemia will reflect V/Q mismatching. Direct metabolic parameters include persistent fever and leukocytosis, hyperglycemia, hypertriglyceridemia, and elevation of blood urea nitrogen (BUN). The increased peripheral demand will result in high cardiac output and low systemic vascular resistance. Other important signs include gastric atony and ileus, continued third spacing and a requirement for fluids, concentrated urine, and encephalopathy. As actual organ dysfunction occurs, serum creatinine will increase, and a pattern consistent with biliary obstruction (elevations of alkaline phosphatase and gamma glutamyltransferase in the serum and bilirubin in the urine) will become evident. These changes herald the onset of MODS. Treatment is complex, primarily supportive, and involves identification and removal of the inciting source.

Transition to shock can take several forms. The most common reflects ongoing, unreplaced fluid losses, such as persistent bleeding. The pattern is similar to that seen in the Ebb phase, with peripheral vasoconstriction, poor perfusion of organs other than brain and heart, and activation of endogenous fluid-conserving mechanisms. Shock may also reflect inadequate fluid administration to a patient with stress and can herald the onset of SIRS/MODS. In these cases, the pattern is different; although there is still a maldistribution of perfusion, this primarily effects the splanchnic circulation. Flow to muscle and skin may be high, cardiac output elevated, and peripheral resistance low.

The treatment of either form of shock starts with the administration of fluids. The next step is identification of the problem;

a septic focus, ongoing bleeding, or some other problem. Inadequately treated shock inevitably results in death.

THE IMPACT OF COMMON PREEXISTING CONDITIONS

Surgical patients present in many different ways. Although trauma victims tend to be young, they often have concurrent problems, particularly substance abuse. Patients who stay in the SICU after elective surgery often have one or more common conditions that can interact with the stress response in an exceedingly important way. In the following, we will examine the effects of three common diseases on the response to surgery, with emphasis on prediction, recognition, and prevention of complications.

Coronary Artery Disease (CAD)

Coronary artery disease is probably the preexisting condition commonly seen in patients admitted to the SICU. Older patients with gastrointestinal, orthopedic, or urologic problems, as well as patients undergoing peripheral vascular surgery frequently have symptomatic or asymptomatic CAD. This condition can effect the stress response in a number of significant ways.

First, CAD should be distiguished from ischemic cardiomyopathy. The latter involves substantial contractile dysfunction at rest and an extremely high risk of death and complications, but is relatively uncommon. In contrast, CAD is common, may be asymptomatic, but most often is characterized by some form of precipitable dysfunction. The most common sign of CAD is angina. Pain may occur after exertion, such as walking. In many cases, a sedentary lifestyle makes it difficult to distinguish exertional pain from rest pain. However, pain that appears to be at rest but occurs in a context when cardiac demand might increase (watching a sporting event, having an argument) is properly considered exertional. In contrast, unprovoked pain at rest or pain that awakens the patient from sleep is by definition unstable angina and demands a thorough work-up. The next discussion will focus on the patient with stable, exertional angina, or asymptomatic CAD, with normal cardiac function.

In CAD, ischemia occurs when substrate demand exceeds substrate supply. Oxygen is believed to be the critical substrate, but that may not be true. Nevertheless, when flow to a region of myocardium is insufficient to meet metabolic needs, ischemia occurs. Persistent ischemia leads to infarction, which in the perioperative period may be highly lethal. This has four obvious implications with respect to perioperative stress. First, myocardial demand will be at its highest at the peak of the stress response, that is, postoperative day 2 to 3. Therefore, the peak incidence of infarction should occur on these days. This prediction is supported by clinical studies. Second, because more extensive procedures require higher energy expenditure and, therefore, higher levels of substrate delivery, the incidence of ischemia should be related to the magnitude of the operation. This is for the most part true, although some procedures (e.g., carotid endarterectomy) have an incidence of ischemia/infarction that would appear to be disproportionate. Third, infarction is something that, especially in the perioperative period, should be avoided at all costs. Finally, strategies that improve myocardial substrate delivery or reduce myocardial work should reduce the incidence of infarction. The caution is that these strategies may be deleterious to function in other organs and may alter outcome on that basis.

Several factors increase myocardial oxygen demand. The principal factor is tachycardia. In addition, hypertension, by increasing wall tension and "strain," also adds to oxygen demand in the outpatient setting. For reasons that are unclear, this is rare in the perioperative period. Oxygen delivery to the myocardium can be decreased by tachycardia (decreased perfusion time), hypertension (increased resistance to flow), hypotension (decreased filling), and anemia (decreased oxygen carrying capacity). This last is especially important, because recent studies indicate an increase in ischemic events with hematocrit less than 27% or hemoglobin concentration less than 9 mg/dL.

With this background, an approach to the patient with CAD can be devised. First, monitoring for ischemia is essential. This often takes the form of continuous ECG monitoring (perhaps with ST trending). Other methods have been used; none is 100% sensitive. It is important to avoid tachycardia. This can be accomplished by:

1. Effectively treating pain
2. Maintaining adequate filling, i.e., avoiding hypotension
3. Maintaining oxygen-carrying capacity
4. Using β-blockade

A recent study indicates improved outcome in patients with CAD who have noncardiac surgery if they began taking atenolol preoperatively and continued to receive the drug postoperatively. Avoiding hypotension and anemia not only helps to prevent tachycardia but also directly improves myocardial substrate delivery.

Therefore, knowledge of the stress response allows us to predict what complications are likely to occur in patients with CAD, when risk is the greatest, and what therapeutic strategies will prevent complications.

Chronic Obstructive Pulmonary Dysfunction (COPD)

Patients with COPD have much in common with patients with CAD, and the two groups often overlap. Therefore, they are often admitted to the SICU after surgery for gastrointestinal, orthopedic, urologic, or vascular problems. In addition, these patients may also need a lung resection. Logically, respiratory insufficiency will be compounded both by the anatomical nature of the surgery and by the demands of the stress response. The stress response increases the requirement for adequate pulmonary function. Although the combination of preexisting hypoxemia, the increase in oxygen consumption, and the obligatory increase in lung water that accompanies hypermetabolism may lead to an apparent oxygen deficit, the key difficulty lies in the excretion of carbon dioxide. Often, hypoxemia is treated easily with supplemental oxygen and early ambulation. CO_2 retention may require ventilatory support.

Knowledge of the stress response allows the prediction that ventilatory failure will occur on postoperative day 2 or 3, as in the patient with CAD. At this point, carbon dioxide production and minute ventilation will be at their highest levels. A compromised patient's ability to excrete CO_2 is likely to fail at this time. Clinically, such a patient will present with agitation, irritability, tachypnea, tachycardia, and hypertension. Eventually, these conditions will give way to lethargy, stupor, declining respiratory rate and, ultimately, respiratory and cardiac arrest. Preventing the patient from arriving in this latter state is essential. In part, this can be accomplished with vigilance and a high index of suspicion. Early ambulation and aggressive pulmonary toilet also benefit the patient. Ideally, all patients with COPD should be ventilated until they passed the peak in VCO_2 and Ve. This is impractical in reality and, therefore, a strategy should be devised to limit prolonged ventilation to only the patients most at risk.

In preparing to manage a patient with known or suspected COPD, it is important to know if the patient has a preoperative defect in oxygenation or ventilation. This allows the development of an algorithm to recognize the patients who are at greatest risk. The patient with baseline hypoxemia usually is adapted. Thus, a realistic goal is to approximate the preoperative PO2. More importantly, it is essential to know if the patient retains CO_2 at baseline. This has ramifications beyond the development of realistic weaning strategies. The patient who retains CO_2 is at risk for pulmonary hypertension, an exceedingly dangerous condition. This patient requires prolonged postoperative observation and perhaps some period of mandatory ventilatory support during which time the CO_2 is allowed to rise to at least preoperative levels.

Thus, knowledge of the stress response, as in the patient with CAD, allows us to predict what complication occurs in the patient with COPD, and when this complication is likely to present. Being aware of the potential complications and instituting preventive measures is sufficient for most patients. High-risk patients, that is, those with CO_2 retention, mandate a more aggressive approach.

Chronic Renal Insufficiency

The patient with chronic renal insufficiency differs from the previous cases. The difficulty in the management of these individuals arises not at the peak of the stress response but at the transition from catabolism to anabolism. Restriction of fluids in these patients is an accepted practice. However, in view of the physiologic changes that accompany surgery, restricting fluids is potentially dangerous. Even dialysis-dependent patients tolerate fluid loads well during the catabolic state because expansion of the extracellular space is a fluid-requiring process that tends to buffer elevations of potassium and acid from endogenous sources. As described in the discussion of prolonged hypercatabolism, failure to administer adequate fluid in this period may contribute to the development of SIRS/MODS. Certainly, hypoperfusion can further compromise renal insufficiency. The problem arises when fluid cannot be mobilized and excreted in the transition to anabolism. The patient may then develop pulmonary edema on a hydrostatic basis, which easily is avoided if anticipated. In the dialysis-dependent patient, scheduling of dialysis should be flexible. The patient with renal insufficiency who is not on dialysis will usually respond to diuretics. Premature administration of diuretics can compromise the stress response, as can over-aggressive removal of water during dialysis. Thus, patients should not be diuresed before the third or fourth postoperative day. This is even more critical for patients who do not have preexisting renal impairment; it is impossible to use diuretics to remove extravascular water that accumulates as a result of a capillary leak. Once again, an understanding of the stress response indicates what the complication may be, when it is likely to occur, and what therapeutic approach to use.

Diabetes Mellitus

Although usually thought of as a disease of glucose metabolism, diabetes is an extremely complicated disorder involving all aspects of metabolism. Nonetheless, given the importance of glucose in the stress response, the effects of diabetes will have profound consequence in the perioperative period. Surgery itself is an insulin-resistant state. Further, the most important function of insulin lies not in altering peripheral uptake of glucose but in limiting hepatic gluconeogenesis. In the postoperative state, glucose levels are elevated by increased release of catecholamines, glucagon, and cortisol. The stimulus for this elevation is multifactorial, but in part, it reflects the increased demand for glucose to fuel white blood cells. Insulin increases as well, primarily in response to elevations in serum glucose levels. Hyperglycemia (levels above 120 mg/dL) is the rule in the postoperative period. The absence of insulin or a relative inability of the liver to respond to insulin and decrease gluconeogenesis, will exacerbate hyperglycemia. This is most pronounced at the peak of the stress response on postoperative day 2 or 3.

The first, most obvious therapeutic option is to limit the administration of exogenous glucose, which does not function to "spare" protein, as occurs in starvation, but simply makes the hyperglycemia more profound. Second, more aggressive hydration is essential to prevent either ketoacidosis or the development of a hyperosmolar state. Finally, insulin should be used cautiously and in the lowest dose possible. A continuous infusion is preferable because it allows better control.

CONCLUSIONS

In this review, we have seen that there is a characteristic, adaptive response to surgical stress. The shock phase of this response can be eliminated with fluid administration, but the hypermetabolic phase, which is essential for wound healing, requires a fixed period to meet the energy demands of repair. The key to management is support of the response and careful observation for deviations from the norm, which can take the form of renewed shock or persistent hypermetabolism. Hypermetabolism often reflects the presence of a persistent inflammatory source and can evolve to become SIRS/MODS. Preexisting diseases will interact with stress, but an understanding of the stress response and the disease will allow one to anticipate what and when a condition is likely to occur and to devise an appropriate therapeutic approach. In this framework, the care of critically ill surgical patients becomes a matter of pattern recognition and early intervention to support the appropriate care and prevent the inappropriate care.

As a final note, the "stress" response is really the response to any inflammatory state or event. Recent data indicates a similar response occurs after uncomplicated myocardial infarction, acute asthma attacks, COPD exacerbations, and nonsurgical infections. Thus, an understanding of this "inflammatory" response may be even more important than initially appreciated.

6

Coronary Care Unit

Steven P. Schulman

ACUTE ISCHEMIC SYNDROMES

Pathophysiology

Acute coronary syndromes (unstable angina, non-Q-wave myocardial infarction, and Q-wave myocardial infarction) are characterized by acute coronary plaque rupture and thrombosis with abrupt decrease in coronary blood flow. Plaque rupture has been demonstrated pathologically in patients dying of unstable angina and myocardial infarction. Importantly, often the nonobstructive, lipid-rich small coronary plaque is prone to rupture. In stable angina patients, the site of a future acute myocardial infarction is unpredictable on the basis of a coronary angiogram. In patients dying of acute myocardial infarction, an inflammatory process in the fibrous coronary plaque at the site of rupture contributes to the acute plaque rupture. This inflammatory process primarily consists of activated macrophages and, to a lesser degree, T lymphocytes that release proteinases and cytokines leading to plaque breakdown and subsequent rupture. Elevated levels of C-reactive protein, an acute-phase reactant and a marker for underlying systemic inflammation, in asymptomatic healthy men predicts risk of future myocardial infarction in asymptomatic healthy men.

In patients presenting within 4 hours of symptom onset with an acute transmural myocardial infarction, 87% of patients had 100% thrombotic occlusion of the infarct-related artery on an emergent coronary angiogram. Because of spontaneous fibrinolysis, the incidence of total thrombotic occlusion decreases with increasing duration of symptoms. Coronary angioscopy has confirmed the presence of red thrombus (often red-cell and fibrin-rich) in patients with an acute transmural infarction. The concept of thrombosis contributing to the pathophysiology of acute myocardial infarction introduced thrombolytic therapy.

In patients with non-Q-wave myocardial infarction and unstable angina, angiography often shows a patent but severely diseased culprit coronary vessel. In contrast to the concentric coronary stenoses often found on catheterization in patients with stable angina, quantitative angiography often shows an eccentric lesion in unstable angina patients. Autopsies have confirmed that angiographic eccentric stenosis is consistent with a ruptured plaque. Transient coronary occlusion from clot formation followed by spontaneous reperfusion likely causes episodes of ischemic pain in these groups of patients. In contrast to patients with Q-wave myocardial infarction, the thrombus on coronary angioscopy in unstable angina patients is often white-grey in appearance (platelet-rich).

Platelet aggregation and thrombosis contribute to the clinical syndromes of unstable angina and myocardial infarction. Patients with unstable angina have elevated levels of thromboxane A2 metabolites and fibrinopeptide A, products of platelet activation and thrombosis respectively. The greater the degree of thrombin activity, the higher the short-term risk of mortality and myocardial infarction in patients with unstable angina. Platelet activation and aggregation lead to the release and accumulation of serotonin and thromboxane A2 in the coronary bed, which results in further platelet aggregation and coronary vasoconstriction. This vasoconstriction can reduce further coronary blood flow and lead to more ischemia. In patients with an acute myocardial infarction, markers of platelet activation significantly increase compared with those in stable angina patients. Platelets from patients with an acute myocardial infarction show a greater amount of adhesion and aggregability compared with platelets from stable angina patients. Furthermore, platelet hyperreactivity measured in patients 3 months after an acute myocardial infarction manifested by spontaneous aggregation independently predicts mortality and recurrent myocardial infarction.

The clinical sequela of a coronary plaque rupture—asymptomatic, unstable angina, non-Q-wave infarction, Q-wave infarction, or sudden death—depends on several local and systemic factors. Local factors include the degree of plaque disruption, plaque composition, and the amount of vasoconstriction. Systemic factors include levels of catecholamines and the degree of platelet and thrombin activation. The onset of a plaque rupture is likely not a random event, triggered to a certain extent by systemic factors, primarily catecholamine concentrations. Thus, the onset of acute myocardial infarction has a circadian variation, peaking in frequency around 9 A.M. with a trough around 11 P.M. This variation is not evident in patients receiving chronic β-adrenergic blocking agents. Other ischemic events have a similar circadian variation, including the onset of stroke, sudden cardiac death, ischemia on continuous electrocardiographic monitoring, and exercise treadmill ischemia. The early morning peak of plasma epinephrine causing an increase in platelet aggregability and vascular tone likely contributes to the circadian variation in ischemic events. Sudden increases in stress, such as severe emotional stress, anger, and unusual levels of exercise, also may trigger acute ischemic events, likely via a similar mechanism.

In addition to the standard risk factors for the development of atherosclerosis, including hypertension, hypercholesterolemia, diabetes, smoking, and family history; other risk factors also may contribute to coronary events. Nonconventional risk factors that may contribute to a hypercoagulable state resulting in premature thrombotic events are listed in Table 6.1.

Table 6.1
Nonconventional Risk Factors for Myocardial Infarction

Hyperhomocystinemia
Angiotensin-converting enzyme DD genotype
Platelet IIb/IIIa receptor polymorphism
Elevated fibrinogen
Elevated plasminogen activator inhibitor
Elevated tissue plasminogen activator antigen
Elevated C-reactive protein
Elevated von Willebrand factor antigen
Chlamydia pneumoniae infection

These risk factors suggest that beyond coronary atheroma, markers of impaired fibrinolysis, inflammation, endothelial injury, and possibly infection may contribute to acute thrombotic events.

UNSTABLE ANGINA

Clinical Classification/Risk Stratification

Unstable angina has several presentations that differ in prognosis. Patients with new onset angina have anginal pain developing within the past 2 months occurring when the patient walks less than two blocks or does minimal activities resulting in a severe limitation to normal activity. Progressive angina describes a patient with previous angina that has progressed in severity in a crescendo pattern leading to severe limitation in normal activity. Rest angina is anginal pain at rest within the last 48 hours. Variant angina is anginal pain not related to physical activity and accompanied by transient ST segment elevation on an electrocardiogram. Patients with postinfarction angina develop ischemic pain 24 hours to 2 weeks after a myocardial infarction.

Patients with postinfarction angina represent the highest risk group for 6 month mortality (11%) and (re)infarction (20%). Patients with rest angina are more likely than those with progressive angina or new onset angina to have recurrent ischemic pain and to require revascularization with either coronary artery bypass surgery or coronary angioplasty. Other predictors of high-risk unstable angina patients for mortality or myocardial infarction include evidence that the ischemia results in hemodynamic compromise. These clinical criteria include pulmonary edema, hypotension, or ischemic mitral regurgitation. Electrocardiographic indicators of increased risk include rest angina with ST segment changes, which predict adverse clinical outcomes of recurrent ischemia, myocardial infarction, or need for revascularization. Rest angina with precordial T-wave inversions also identifies patients with a high risk for myocardial infarction and mortality as a result of critical proximal left anterior descending coronary artery stenosis. Finally, in patients with unstable angina and a non-Q-wave myocardial infarction, an elevated troponin level on admission increases the risk of short-term mortality compared with patients with acute ischemic syndromes and normal admission troponin levels. Patients with unstable angina and elevated troponin levels likely have suffered small areas of myocardial necrosis from transient coronary occlusion and are at risk for further ischemic damage.

Medical Therapy

The initial stabilization of the patient with cardiac ischemia includes assurance of a secure and stable airway and maintenance of breathing. Medical therapy goals include stabilizing with relief of pain and ischemia and developing a treatment plan based on risk stratification. Therapy may include heparin, aspirin, β-adrenergic receptor blockers, nitroglycerin, and calcium-channel blockers. If medical therapy does not control ischemic pain, consider urgent coronary angiography with revascularization and placement of an intra-aortic balloon pump to improve coronary perfusion and relieve ischemia.

Based on the pathophysiology of unstable angina, the cornerstone of therapy is antithrombotic and antiplatelet therapy. Heparin is more beneficial than aspirin alone in preventing myocardial infarction in this patient group. However, recurrent ischemia occurs in about 15% of patients with unstable angina who initially were stabilized with heparin therapy. This rebound ischemia is likely from a hypercoagulable state produced from a transient rebound in thrombin activity after heparin cessation in patients with acute coronary syndromes. Platelet inhibition induced by aspirin may prevent reactivation of an acute ischemic syndrome after heparin cessation in unstable angina patients. Aspirin therapy also offers long-term protection from recurrent acute ischemia and mortality in patients admitted with unstable angina. The platelet antagonist ticlopidine can reduce mortality and nonfatal myocardial infarction in unstable angina patients.

Platelet aggregation is mediated exclusively by the platelet fibrinogen receptor glycoprotein (GP) IIb/IIIa. The receptor's fibrinogen binding is the final common pathway leading to platelet aggregation and thrombus formation. After plaque rupture, the exposure of blood to the adhesive vessel wall proteins as collagen and von Willebrand Factor result in platelets adhering to the vessel wall. After adhesion, a conformational change occurs to platelet

IIb/IIIa receptors causing platelet activation. Platelets now adhere with high affinity to fibrinogen and von Willebrand Factor causing platelet aggregation and thrombosis. Although aspirin therapy benefits patients with acute ischemic syndromes of unstable angina and acute myocardial infarction, it is a weak inhibitor of platelet aggregation. Despite permanent inhibition of cyclooxygenase activity, aspirin does not prevent other agonist-mediated platelet activation and aggregation, such as thrombin or serotonin. Several inhibitors of the glycoprotein IIb/IIIa platelet receptor have been developed that limit platelet aggregation to a greater degree than aspirin therapy and may be useful in treating unstable angina patients. Clinical trials are evaluating GP IIb/IIIa receptor inhibitors in patients with unstable angina.

New antithrombotic agents for patients with acute ischemic syndromes have been developed because of several disadvantages with the use of standard unfractionated heparin, including ineffectiveness against clot-bound thrombin, inactivation by plasma proteins, and thrombocytopenia. Hirudin is a small peptide that is a direct inhibitor of thrombin, can inhibit clot-bound thrombin, is not inactivated by platelet factor 4, and does not cause thrombocytopenia. The effectiveness of recombinant hirudin compared with that of heparin in acute coronary syndromes was evaluated in the Global Use of Strategies to Open Occluded Coronary Arteries (GUSTO) IIb Study. The 30-day primary end-points of death or nonfatal myocardial infarction was not different in patients randomly given hirudin (8.3%) compared with heparin (9.1%). Another group of antithrombotic agents, low molecular weight heparins, is being evaluated for the treatment of unstable angina. Low molecular weight heparins inhibit thrombin as well as thrombin production, has a greater bioavailability, a longer half-life, and a more predictable dose response than unfractionated heparin. Other potential benefits of low molecular weight heparin include less thrombocytopenia and it is given subcutaneously, so it has potential outpatient and chronic uses. Preliminary data of patients with unstable angina and non-Q-wave myocardial infarctions suggest that, compared with unfractionated heparin, low molecular weight heparin for at least 48 hours reduces the composite endpoint of death, myocardial infarction, or recurrent angina. Trials investigating acute and chronic low molecular weight heparin in unstable angina and non-Q-wave myocardial infarction are in progress.

The effects of thrombolytic therapy in patients with unstable angina or a non-Q-wave myocardial infarction was evaluated in the Thrombolysis in Myocardial Infarction (TIMI) IIIb Study. In addition to standard therapy with aspirin, heparin, and anti-ischemic therapy, patients were randomly given 0.8 mg/kg of tissue plasminogen activator versus placebo. Although 6-week mortality was similar in the two groups, the incidence of myocardial infarction was greater in patients who received thrombolytic therapy compared with those who received placebo.

Revascularization

Unstable angina patients who present with a high-risk clinical profile should be considered for early cardiac catheterization and revascularization with percutaneous balloon angioplasty techniques or coronary artery bypass surgery. Early revascularization in this group of patients is because of the considerable risk of myocardial infarction and/or death over the next several months with continued medical therapy. Patients with continued or recurrent ischemic rest pain despite aspirin, heparin, β-adrenergic receptor blockade, and nitroglycerin should be considered for urgent cardiac catheterization and revascularization. Patients with postinfarction angina with ischemic ST changes are a high-risk group who also should be considered for revascularization. Patients with postinfarction angina and an ejection fraction less than 50% who underwent angioplasty have improved survival with a patent infarct vessel compared with those with a closed infarct vessel. The Thrombolysis in Myocardial Infarction IIIB Clinical Trial addressed whether routine invasive evaluation for patients with unstable angina or a non-Q-wave myocardial infarction should be considered. This study suggests that routine cardiac catheterization with revascularization is not required in all patients with unstable angina. The Veterans Administration Study evaluated the influence of coronary artery bypass surgery on survival in unstable angina patients. This study suggests that unstable angina patients who are candidates for surgery and have triple vessel coronary artery disease, especially with impairment of left ventricular function, should be considered for coronary artery bypass surgery.

NON-Q-WAVE MYOCARDIAL INFARCTION

Management of patients with non-Q-wave myocardial infarction is similar to that of patients with unstable angina, including therapy with aspirin and heparin, β-adrenergic receptor blockade and nitroglycerin. Patients with non-Q-wave infarction have a higher recurrent ischemic rate, yet routine cardiac catheterization and revascularization does not reduce mortality or recurrent myocardial infarction. Preliminary data from the Veterans Administration non-Q-wave Infarction Strategies in Hospital Trial suggest that invasive evaluation should be reserved for patients with non-Q-wave infarction who are at high risk for recurrent ischemic events or mortality (Table 6.2).

Q-WAVE MYOCARDIAL INFARCTION

Risk Stratification

Risk stratification for patients with acute myocardial infarction must begin immediately upon presentation. Immediate decisions concerning eligibility for thrombolytic therapy or primary angioplasty are necessary. Patients who receive thrombolytic therapy need to be further risk stratified according to whether they have achieved clinical reperfusion (low risk) or need to be considered for emergent rescue angioplasty. Further identification of high-risk patient subgroups can be determined by clinical history, physical examination, and the admission electrocardiogram (Table 6.3).

Although there is a great deal of data that suggest patients with an acute myocardial infarction with any of these characteristics are

Table 6.2
Indications for Revascularization in Patients with Unstable Angina

Recurrent/refractory ischemia
Postinfarction angina
High-risk presentation, i.e., pulmonary edema
Exercise test positive for ischemia
Known/suspected triple vessel disease with impaired LV function

Table 6.3
High-Risk Patient Subsets with Q-Wave Myocardial Infarction

Clinical: Increasing patient age, history of prior myocardial infarction, history of congestive heart failure, postinfarction angina
Examination: Hypotension, rales, S3 gallop, mitral regurgitation, tachycardia
Electrocardiogram: Increasing number of leads with ST segment elevation, precordial ST segment depression with an inferior infarction, right ventricular infarction, inferior ST segment depression with an anterior infarct, atrial arrhythmias or sinus tachycardia, monomorphic ventricular tachycardia

at increased risk for early mortality, there is a lot less data that demonstrates that early cardiac catheterization with angioplasty or coronary artery bypass surgery reduces these risks. Patients with postinfarction angina should have early coronary angiography because of increased risk of further ischemic damage. Those patients with impaired left ventricular function likely have improved survival with revascularization. Similarly, patients with a prior myocardial infarction, a history of heart failure, or evidence on examination of hemodynamic compromise and/or heart failure often have triple vessel coronary artery disease and left ventricular dysfunction, a subset of postinfarction patients who will have a survival advantage with coronary artery bypass surgery. Early cardiac catheterization should therefore be considered in this group.

MEDICAL THERAPY

Antiplatelet Therapy

Aspirin in a dose of 160 mg to 325 mg should be given to all patients with acute myocardial infarction. The initial dose should be chewed if possible for rapid absorption. The Second International Trial of Infarct Survival (ISIS-2) demonstrated a 23% reduction in 35-day mortality in those patients randomly taking 160 mg of aspirin therapy. Aspirin combined with streptokinase had a synergistic benefit on 35-day mortality compared with placebo. Significant reductions in short-term reinfarction and stroke were also demonstrated with aspirin therapy. Since in vitro spontaneous platelet aggregation is a reliable predictor of 5-year recurrent myocardial infarction and mortality, aspirin therapy should be continued long term in survivors of acute myocardial infarction.

Thrombolytic Therapy

The Fibrinolytic Therapy Trialists' Collaborative Group performed a meta-analysis of nine randomized trials of fibrinolytic therapy versus control showing a 35-day mortality of 9.6% in the thrombolytic arm versus an 11.5% mortality in the control arm, representing an 18% reduction in mortality with thrombolytic therapy. The mortality based on the presenting electrocardiogram is shown in Table 6.4. Patients with inferior ST segment elevation benefit from thrombolytic therapy to a lesser extent, but those with ST segment depression do not benefit. The greater number of leads with ST segment elevation or the greater amount of ST segment elevation, the larger the infarction, and the greater the benefit from thrombolysis. Furthermore, patients presenting with ST segment elevation in the precordial leads with inferior ST segment depression are at greater risk than those without inferior ST segment changes and benefit more from thrombolytic therapy. Similarly, patients with ST segment elevation in the inferior leads with associated precordial ST segment depression (inferoposterior injury) also benefit more from thrombolytic therapy than those patients with solely inferior ST segment elevation.

Limiting the time to achieving coronary artery reperfusion is critical to maximizing the number of lives saved with thrombolytic therapy. Significant reductions in short-term mortality are seen with thrombolytic therapy given within 12 hours of symptom onset of an acute myocardial infarction. Although treating patients who arrive within 12 to 24 hours of symptoms does not result in a significant reduction in 35-day mortality, thrombolytic therapy should be considered for those patients who have persistent ischemic pain and a large area of ischemic myocardium at risk as determined by

Table 6.4
Effect of Thrombolytic Therapy on 35-Day Mortality Based on ECG

	Fibrinolytic (%)	Control (%)
Bundle branch block	18.7	23.6
Anterior ST elevation	13.2	16.9
Inferior ST elevation	7.5	8.4
ST depression	15.2	13.8

multiple leads with ST segment elevation. There is an inverse linear relationship between absolute reduction in 35-day mortality and time from symptom onset to receiving thrombolytic therapy in patients with ST segment elevation or bundle branch block on the electrocardiogram. For every hour delay from the onset of symptoms to receiving thrombolytic therapy, there is a reduction in 1.6 lives saved per every 1,000 acute infarct patients treated with thrombolytic therapy. For every 30-minute delay in receiving thrombolytic therapy, infarct size increases 1% as determined by thallium scintigraphy scanning. The critical need to achieve reperfusion as early as possible has been emphasized in studies of patients who have received prehospital thrombolytic therapy. Patients who received thrombolytic therapy within 60 to 90 minutes of symptom onset often have no scintigraphic evidence of an infarction with an associated in-hospital mortality of only 1 to 2%.

The high mortality of acute myocardial infarction in the elderly, suggests that this group of patients may benefit from more aggressive therapies. Even after adjusting for the facts that older patients with infarction more likely have nondiagnostic electrocardiograms or a non-Q-wave myocardial infarction, as well as arrive later to the hospital than younger patients, older patients who are candidates for thrombolytic therapy are less likely to receive it.

Contraindications to thrombolytic therapy are listed in Table 6.5. The main risks are bleeding, with the greatest concern being intracerebral hemorrhage with thrombolysis. Fibrinolytic therapy is associated with a stroke rate of 1.2% of patients treated with thrombolytic versus 0.8% of controls. The excess of strokes with therapy occurs on day 1, the majority of these early neurologic events are attributed to intracranial hemorrhage. Risk factors for the development of intracranial hemorrhage include prior cerebrovascular disease, older age, low body weight, elevated diastolic blood pressure, history of hypertension, and elevated systolic blood pressure. Patients who are ineligible for therapy with thrombolytics have a high short-term mortality from their myocardial infarction, estimated at 15 to 21%.

The Gruppo Italiano per lo Studio della Sopravvivenze nell'Infarto Miocardico (GISSI-2)/International trial randomized nearly 21,000 patients presenting within 6 hours of ischemic chest

Table 6.5
Contraindications to Thrombolytic Therapy Use

Absolute contraindications
- Cerebral vascular accident within 1 year
- Cerebral hemorrhage at any time
- Known intracranial neoplasm
- Suspected aortic dissection
- Acute pericarditis
- Active GI/GU bleeding

Relative contraindications
- Uncontrolled hypertension (BP >180/110 mm Hg)
- Bleeding diathesis
- Recent GI/GU bleeding (within 2–4 weeks)
- History of chronic severe hypertension
- Distant cerebral vascular accident or any intracerebral pathology
- Major trauma within 2–4 weeks including major surgery or head trauma
- Current use of anticoagulants
- CPR > 10 minutes
- Pregnancy

pain and meeting electrocardiographic criteria for thrombolytic therapy to receive 1.5 million units of SK over 1 hour or 100 mg of t-PA over 3 hours. All patients received aspirin. In a second randomization, patients received either subcutaneous heparin, 12,500 units twice daily or placebo beginning 12 hours after thrombolytic therapy was initiated. The Third International Study of Infarct Survival (ISIS-3) randomized more than 41,000 patients presenting within 24 hours of symptom onset of suspected acute myocardial infarction to receive either SK, t-PA, or APSAC. All patients received aspirin. A second randomization in this study also evaluated 12,500 units twice daily of subcutaneous heparin versus placebo beginning 4 hours after thrombolytic therapy initiation. In both the GISSI-2 and ISIS-3 studies, there was an excess in strokes in patients randomized to tissue plasminogen activator. This excess was because of an increase in intracerebral hemorrhage, particularly in the elderly. The use of high-dose subcutaneous heparin did not result in a reduction in 35-day mortality. The Global Utilization of Streptokinase and Tissue Plasminogen Activator for Occluded Coronary Arteries (GUSTO-1) Study randomized 41,021 patients with acute myocardial infarction, presenting within 6 hours to one of four regimens:

1. Front-loaded t-PA (15 mg bolus, 0.75 mg/kg over 30 minutes, not to exceed 50 mg; then 0.5 mg/kg over 1 hour, not to exceed 35 mg) with full-dose intravenous heparin
2. 1.5 MU SK over 60 minutes plus 12,500 units subcutaneous heparin twice daily
3. 1.5 MU SK over 60 minutes with full-dose intravenous heparin
4. 1.0 mg/kg t-PA over 60 minutes, not to exceed 90 mg, plus 1.0 MU SK, plus full-dose intravenous heparin

All patients received aspirin. Thirty-day mortality was reduced significantly in patients randomized to the front-loaded t-PA regimen (Table 6.6). An excess of total stroke and hemorrhagic strokes was again seen in the t-PA regimen, although the combined end point of death and nonfatal disabling stroke was still significantly lower in this group.

The averaged comparison in these three large trials between t-PA and SK for the end point of 30-day stroke or death suggests no significant difference between the two agents. A greater number of lives will be saved with timely, full use of any of the approved thrombolytic agents in acute myocardial infarction.

The critical importance of establishing coronary arterial patency with thrombolytic therapy was emphasized in the GUSTO angiographic substudy. In this study, no matter which agent was used, 30-day mortality was lowest, 4.4%, in patients with normal flow in the infarct vessel (TIMI III) at 90 minutes; intermediate, 7.4%, in patients with complete vessel opacification but delayed

Table 6.6
Major Clinical Outcomes in the GUSTO-I Trial

	t-PA+I.V. Hep (%)	SK+S.Q. Hep (%)	SK+I.V. Hep (%)	t-pA+SK (%)
30-day death	6.3	7.2	7.4	7 0
30-day death+ nonfatal disabling stroke	6.9	7.7	7.9	7.6

t-PA, tissue plasminogen activator; *SK,* streptokinase; *HEP,* heparin filling or washout (TIMI II) at 90 minutes; and worst, 8.9%, with lack of patency (TIMI 0,1) at 90 minutes. TIMI (Thrombolysis in Myocardial Infarction) grade flow also correlated well with left ventricular function, with patients with TIMI III flow having the best left ventricular function recovery. The mortality benefit of t-PA compared with SK in the GUSTO trial was because of the improved TIMI III flow at 90 minutes.

Antithrombotic Therapy

Before the known benefits and routine use of aspirin and fibrinolytics in acute myocardial infarction, a meta-analysis of studies comparing intravenous heparin with control show a reduction in death, stroke, and pulmonary embolism with an increase in major bleeding in patients randomized to full doses of heparin. Currently, in therapy for acute myocardial infarction with aspirin and thrombolytic therapy, the ISIS-3 and GISSI-2 trials evaluated high-dose subcutaneous heparin versus placebo. Thirty-five day mortality was not decreased in patients who received subcutaneous heparin plus aspirin compared with those who received aspirin alone; however, during the duration of subcutaneous heparin therapy, mortality was slightly reduced. Bleeding also increased in the heparin-treated patients. Intravenous heparin is beneficial in patients with acute myocardial infarction treated with the fibrin-specific agent, t-PA, which causes less of a systemic lytic state and has a shorter half-life than SK. In patients with acute myocardial infarction treated with t-PA, patency of the infarct vessel at 18 hours is significantly higher for patients treated with full-dose intravenous heparin compared with those treated with low-dose aspirin alone. Patients treated with t-PA should receive intravenous heparin for 48 to 72 hours with a goal activated partial thromboplastin time (aPTT) of 50 to 75 seconds. Attempts to use more aggressive levels of anticoagulation (aPTT) up to 90 seconds with heparin leads to an unacceptably high risk of intracerebral hemorrhage. Finally, unless contraindicated, 7500 units of subcutaneous heparin twice daily should be administered to all patients with infarction who are not receiving intravenous heparin until they are able to walk to prevent deep vein thrombosis and pulmonary emboli. In patients at high risk for intracardiac thrombi (large infarction, anterior wall infarction, atrial arrhythmias, and prior embolic event), full-dose heparin should be considered unless contraindicated.

Beta-Adrenergic Receptor Blockade

Beta-adrenergic receptor (β) blockade has many benefits for the treatment of acute myocardial infarction. Acutely, β-blocker therapy will lower heart rate and blood pressure, resulting in decreased chest pain and infarct size. The First International Study of Infarct Survival (ISIS-1) was largest randomized trial of intravenous followed by oral β-blocker therapy in acute myocardial infarction. This study, performed in the prethrombolytic era, randomized 16,027 patients with a suspected acute myocardial infarction within 12 hours of symptom onset to intravenous, followed by oral atenolol for 7 days versus control. The main end point, 7-day vascular mortality, was significantly reduced 15% in the group receiving β-blocker therapy. All the mortality benefit was on the first day of therapy; thereafter, the mortality curves were parallel. The combined end point of death, ventricular fibrillation, and recurrent myocardial infarction also was reduced significantly by β-blocker therapy. In a meta-analysis of the 28 randomized trials of intravenous β-blocker therapy in acute myocardial infarction, short-term mortality, reinfarction, and ventricular fibrillation are reduced significantly with therapy.

The TIMI II-B Study determined the benefits of acute β-blocker therapy in patients who have received thrombolytic therapy, aspirin, and heparin. Patients were randomized to immediate intravenous metoprolol followed by oral metoprolol versus oral metoprolol begun on day 6. The primary end point of this trial, predischarge ejection fraction, was not different between the two groups. Secondary clinical differences were noted at 6 days and 6 weeks, but not at 1 year, including reduced nonfatal reinfarction in the immediate β-blocker group. Recurrent chest pain also decreased in the immediate therapy group. Because of a reduction in blood pressure with immediate β-blocker therapy, intracranial hemorrhage was less likely to occur in this group of patients.

These studies demonstrate the benefits of β-blocker therapy in acute myocardial infarction. The relative contraindications to acute intravenous β-blocker therapy are shown in Table 6.7.

Table 6.7
Relative Contraindications to β-Blocker Therapy

- Resting heart rate < 55/min
- Systolic blood pressure < 100 mmHg
- Cardiogenic shock or rales $> 1/3$
- PR interval > 0.24 second
- Second or third degree heart block
- Significant bronchospasm or chronic obstructive lung disease

Angiotensin-Converting Enzyme (ACE) Inhibition

Infarct expansion, the pathologic stretching and thinning of the infarct zone, is a frequent complication of acute myocardial infarction, resulting in an increased risk of congestive heart failure and mortality within hours to days of a myocardial infarction. After stretching and thinning of the infarct zone, long-term increases in cardiac volume are the result of a progressive decline in noninfarct zone function. Clinical predictors of infarct expansion include Q-wave myocardial infarction, anterior location, large infarct size, and an occluded infarct vessel. A patent infarct vessel, even without salvaging myocardium, may result in a decrease in infarct expansion and subsequent aneurysm formation.

In patients with an acute Q-wave myocardial infarction, treatment with angiotensin-converting enzyme (ACE) inhibitors limit the increases in end-diastolic and systolic volumes and improves ejection fraction from 1 to 12 months after the infarction.

ACE inhibitors limit infarct expansion and, therefore, reduce mortality and morbidity in patients after an acute myocardial infarction. Several randomized placebo-controlled trials of ACE inhibitors in postinfarct patients at high risk (ejection fraction less than 40%, clinical heart failure, nonthrombolyzed anterior wall myocardial infarctions, echocardiographic wall motion index abnormality less than 1.2, which corresponds to an ejection fraction of less than 35%) demonstrate a 20% reduction in mortality in the group randomized to ACE inhibitors. A summary of several of these trials is shown in Table 6.8. Exclusion criteria for these trials included renal failure (creatinine greater than 2.5 mg/dL), systolic blood pressure less than 100 mmHg, need for ACE inhibitor for severe heart failure, or intolerance or previous side effects to ACE inhibitors.

Two large infarct trials determined whether ACE-inhibitor

Table 6.8
Randomized Trials of ACE Inhibitors in High-Risk Infarct Patients

	N	Inclusion Criteria	Study Drug Initiation	Follow-Up	Mortality ACE/Placebo (%)
SAVE	2231	MI/EF ≤ 40%	Day 3–16	Mean 42 mo	20.4/24.6
AIRE	2006	MI/CHF	Day 3–10	Mean 15 mo	17/23
SMILE	1566	ANT MI (nonthrombolyzed)	Day 1	Mean 12 mo	4.9/6.5
TRACE	1749	MI/WMI ≤ 1.2	Day 3–7	24–50 mo	34.7/42.3

SAVE, Survival and Ventricular Enlargement Trial; *AIRE,* Acute Infarction Ramipril Efficacy Trial; *SMILE,* Survial of Myocardial Infarction: Long-term Evaluation Trial; *TRACE,* Trandolapril Cardiac Evaluation Study; *MI,* myocardial infarction; *EF,* ejection fraction; *CHF,* clinical heart failure; *ANT,* anterior; *WMI,* wall motion index; *mo,* months

therapy benefits all patients arriving with suspected myocardial infarction within 24 hours of admission. The GISSI-3 trial randomized patients who presented with symptoms of acute myocardial infarction within 24 hours to ACE-inhibitor therapy versus placebo for 6 weeks. Also, patients were randomly assigned to nitroglycerin therapy or control. Mortality at 6 weeks was reduced from 7.1% in the control group to 6.3% in the ACE-inhibitor group. Mortality and left ventricular dysfunction were reduced 10% by echocardiography. The Fourth International Study of Infarct Survival randomized ACE-inhibitor therapy or placebo for 1 month to 58,050 infarct patients who presented within 24 hours. Patients also were randomized to nitrates and/or intravenous magnesium. Thirty-five day mortality was reduced from 7.7 to 7.2% in the ACE-inhibitor treated patients. The mortality benefit on the first hospital day suggests a potential algorithm for use of ACE inhibitors including starting therapy for all patients with acute myocardial infarction without a contraindication on the day of admission. In patients with clinical heart failure, anterior wall infarction, or left ventricular dysfunction (ejection fraction less than 40%), ACE-inhibitor therapy should continue indefinitely. In patients with preserved left ventricular function and no clinical heart failure or need for ACE-inhibitor therapy to treat hypertension, the small absolute benefit suggests that the ACE inhibitor need not be continued for the long term.

For patients who are intolerant to ACE-inhibitor therapy because of cough, angiotensin II type 1 receptor antagonists may be an alternative therapy.

Primary Angioplasty

A series of patients presenting with chest pain up to 6 to 12 hours duration and the electrocardiogram demonstrating acute ST-segment elevation have received primary angioplasty. These series show that direct angioplasty in acute transmural myocardial infarction is safe and results in a high level of reperfusion with a low in-hospital mortality and complication rate. These promising results in acute myocardial infarction lead to several randomized trials comparing primary angioplasty with thrombolytic therapy in acute ST-segment elevation myocardial infarction (Table 6.9).

Primary angioplasty should be considered for those patients who arrive within 12 hours of symptom onset of an ST-segment elevation myocardial infarction to a hospital center that performs a high volume number of angioplasty cases at a time when the "door-to-balloon" time is minimal. In centers without the ability to perform angioplasty, without highly trained personnel, or with a delay in mobilizing an angioplasty team, thrombolytic therapy is an excellent life-saving alternative.

The following patients also should be considered for primary

Table 6.9
Primary Angioplasty vs. Thrombolytic Therapy in AMI

	N	Inclusion	Thrombolytic	Mortality PTCA/ LYTIC (%)	ReMI PTCA/ LYTIC (%)	F/U
PAMI	395	CP within 12 hr/STõ↑	t-PA/3 hr	2.6/6.5	2.6/6.5	Hosp
Netherlands	301	CP within 6 hr/STõ↑	SK	2/7	1/10	Hosp
GUSTO IIb	1138	CP within 12 hr/STõ↑	t-PA/1.5 hr	57/7	4.4/6.5	30 d

PAMI, Primary Angioplasty in Myocardial Infarction; *GUSTO,* Global Use of Strategies to Open Occluded Coronary Arteries in Acute Coronary Syndromes; *CP,* chest pain; *AMI,* acute myocardial infarction; *SK,* streptokinase; *t-PA,* tissue plasminogen activator; *PTCA,* percutaneous transluminal coronary angioplasty; *Lytic,* thrombolytic; *F/U,* follow-up; *Hosp,* hospital; *d,* day angioplasty for acute ST-segment elevation myocardial infarction; although there is less data whether this procedure results in better outcome than standard medical therapy. These patients include the following:

1. High-risk patients ineligible for thrombolytic therapy. There is no randomized data of primary angioplasty compared with standard medical therapy. In series of patients undergoing primary angioplasty, those who are thrombolytic ineligible have a substantially higher in-hospital mortality (14%) than those who are thrombolytic eligible (3%).
2. Patients in cardiogenic shock

Angioplasty After Thrombolytic Therapy

Routine immediate cardiac catheterization with balloon angioplasty in patients who have received thrombolytic therapy and reperfused is associated with a higher complication rate and need for urgent coronary artery bypass surgery than elective balloon angioplasty. The TIMI IIb trial compared an invasive and conservative strategy in 3262 patients who have received thrombolytic therapy for an acute myocardial infarction. This trial demonstrated that routine cardiac catheterization with attempted revascularization does not prolong survival or prevent myocardial infarction in patients who have received thrombolytic therapy for acute myocardial infarction. Second, a large number of patients treated conservatively have recurrent ischemia, which should be treated with cardiac catheterization and revascularization. Finally, this approach results in an excellent long-term survival in these patients.

There is only limited data and controversy concerning rescue angioplasty, which is proceeding to emergent cardiac catheterization and angioplasty in patients who have not reperfused after thrombolytic therapy. Although thrombolytic therapy results in TIMI II and III flow in approximately 80% of patients, it is often difficult at the bedside to determine who has not reperfused. Clinical parameters such as persistent chest pain and persistent ST segment elevation suggest failure of thrombolytic therapy. The largest randomized trial of rescue angioplasty involved 150 patients who received thrombolytic therapy for an acute anterior wall infarction and did not reperfuse with TIMI grade 0–1 flow down the left anterior descending. Patients were randomized to immediate angioplasty versus conservative therapy. The primary end point of this trial, ejection fraction on day 30, was not different between the two groups. Rescue angioplasty was beneficial in the secondary end point of death or congestive heart failure at 30 days, although the confidence intervals were large in this small trial. One should consider emergent cardiac catheterization and rescue angioplasty in patients who clinically have not reperfused with thrombolytic therapy and have a large area of jeopardized myocardium, including anterior myocardial infarction, infero-posterior myocardial infarction, or hemodynamic compromise.

SUBGROUPS OF PATIENTS WITH ACUTE INFARCTION

Cardiogenic Shock

Cardiogenic shock syndrome occurs in approximately 8% of all patients with a myocardial infarction. This incidence, nor a mortality rate of 70 to 80%, has not changed over the last 20 years even with the introduction of thrombolytic therapy. The majority of coronary care unit mortality is from patients with cardiogenic shock. Clinically, the syndrome results from the inability of the heart to deliver adequate flow to the tissues in the presence of elevated filling pressures. Patients are hypotensive with blood pressures less than 90 mmHg or 30 mmHg below baseline with hypoperfusion with decreased urine output and vasoconstriction. Also, patients often have pulmonary congestion. Hemodynamics from pulmonary artery catheterization include a decreased cardiac index of less than 2.2 L/min/m^2 with an elevated pulmonary capillary wedge pressure of more than 18 mmHg. The causes of cardiogenic shock from acute myocardial infarction include the following:

1. Loss of a critical amount of left ventricular myocardium, often more than or equal to 40% either from a very large single infarction or the cumulative loss of functioning myocardium from multiple infarctions
2. Right ventricular infarction, complicating an acute inferior wall infarct
3. Acute mitral regurgitation

4. Acute ventricular septal defect
5. Free-wall rupture

In a large series of patients with cardiogenic shock, the median time for diagnosis of shock is 8 hours after onset of acute myocardial infarction; few patients have shock on arrival to the hospital. After the myocardial infarction, shock usually develops after infarct expansion, activation of the sympathetic nervous system and renin angiotensin system, use of vasopressors, and, possibly, ischemia in other areas. This response leads to the downward spiral of progressive left ventricular dysfunction and hypotension. Rapid clinical assessment is imperative in this patient group. Further evaluation should include an echocardiogram to assess left ventricular function, and to determine any mechanical etiology to cardiogenic shock, including a ventricular septal defect, ruptured papillary muscle, free-wall rupture, or a large pericardial effusion. Most patients will require pulmonary artery catheterization to determine and optimize filling pressures and to measure the hemodynamic response to therapy. Finally, although intra-aortic balloon counterpulsation does not change mortality in cardiogenic shock, it can provide hemodynamic support as a bridge to more definitive therapy, such as balloon angioplasty or coronary artery bypass surgery.

The use of reperfusion and revascularization in patients in cardiogenic shock from an acute myocardial infarction is uncertain. In a small subgroup of patients with cardiogenic shock enrolled in the GISSI trial, a 30-day mortality rate was similar in the streptokinase and control treated patients. Angiographic data suggest that the use of thrombolytic therapy in patients in cardiogenic shock has a low reperfusion rate. The efficacy of balloon angioplasty and, to a lesser extent, coronary artery bypass surgery has been reported in several series of patients. Compared with historical control subjects, short- and long-term mortality in revascularized patients is favorable. Although these studies are encouraging, there is considerable selection bias in which patients with cardiogenic shock are selected for cardiac catheterization. In an international registry of patients with cardiogenic shock from a myocardial infarction, patients selected for cardiac catheterization are younger and have a lower in-hospital mortality rate than those who do not undergo cardiac catheterization even if they do not have revascularization.

Mechanical Complications

Free-wall rupture is often a life-ending complication of acute myocardial infarction manifesting as acute electromechanical dissociation. Risks for free-wall rupture include a first infarct, increasing age, and transmural infarction. In the GISSI-2 trial, the cause of death was evaluated in all enrolled patients with a first transmural myocardial infarction treated with thrombolytic therapy. Cardiac rupture was revealed in 65% of autopsies. The incidence of cardiac rupture increased with increasing age. As high as 86% of autopsied hearts of patients more than 70 years old had free-wall rupture. Although cardiac rupture is almost always associated with immediate death, patients rarely survive attributed to pseudo aneurysm formation from pericardial inflammation. Clinically, patients with subacute rupture present with a postinfarct picture of shock and pericardial tamponade, requiring immediate evaluation and surgical management. Selected patients treated medically have experienced long-term survival.

Acute ventricular septal defects occur in approximately 2% of transmural infarcts, usually within 72 hours after the infarction. Clinical findings include acute hemodynamic deterioration with heart failure often with hypotension, and a new holosystolic murmur along the left sternal border. Pulmonary artery catheterization shows elevated filling pressures often with "V" waves. These hemodynamics are similar to acute mitral regurgitation. Patients with a ventricular septal defect can be distinguished from acute mitral regurgitation by measuring oxygen saturations with right ventricular catheterization; those with a ventricular septal defect have an oxygen saturation step-up from the right atrium to the right ventricle and pulmonary artery. Echocardiography often confirms the septal defect with evidence of left to right ventricular flow by Doppler. Patients with hemodynamic compromise have a nearly 100% mortality without urgent surgical intervention. Early cardiac catheterization with intra-aortic balloon support to define the coronary anatomy and site of rupture is often necessary in patients with an acute ventricular septal defect. Although early surgical mortality is high, these patients do poorly without surgical repair. Long-term follow-up in these patients who survive their surgeries show a reasonable survival free of heart failure.

Similar to the presentation with an acute ventricular septal defect, acute mitral regurgitation can cause fulminant shock in a previously stable patient. Patients with this syndrome often present with an inferior myocardial infarction because the posteromedial papillary muscle is supplied by end branches of the posterior descending coronary artery. Acute mitral regurgitation with pulmonary edema and often with hemodynamic compromise may be from rupture of the posteromedial papillary muscle, rupture of chordae tendineae supporting the mitral leaflets, or dysyngery of the area of myocardium supporting the anterior or posterior papillary muscle, resulting in incomplete mitral leaflet closure and mitral regurgitation. The patient with acute mitral regurgitation is often in extremis, requiring mechanical ventilation. Q-wave inferior myocardial infarction usually is present. The murmur of mitral regurgitation may be soft, brief, or absent because of the rapid equalization of pressures between the ventricle and atrium. The diagnosis must be considered in patients who acutely decompensate with pulmonary edema. Echocardiography often shows preserved left ventricular function, and a flail mitral leaflet may be present. Patients with acute mitral regurgitation with hemodynamic compromise need emergent cardiac catheterization often with intra-aortic balloon support to define coronary anatomy. Although emergent angioplasty may improve ischemia-related mitral regurgitation, emergent surgery with coronary artery bypass grafting and mitral valve repair or replacement is often required for a mechanically flailed mitral valve from acute inferior myocardial infarction. Although surgical mortality is high, prognosis with medical therapy is dismal.

Right Ventricular Infarction

Right ventricular free-wall branches usually come off the right coronary artery; therefore, right ventricular infarction occurs with a proximal right coronary artery occlusion. The usual setting of right ventricular infarction is with an acute ST-segment elevation inferior myocardial infarction. The fact that only 15% of acute inferior infarctions clinically present with right ventricular infarction is because the thinner walled right ventricle (which also gets collateral blood flow from the left coronary) has a better oxygen supply:demand ratio than the left ventricle and, therefore, is less likely to infarct.

All patients presenting with an acute inferior myocardial infarction should have right-sided precordial leads performed in addition to the routine electrocardiogram. In a series of 200 consecutive acute inferior myocardial infarctions, diagnostic ST-segment elevation in V4R was observed in 54% of patients. Comparing ST-segment elevation in V4R with autopsy, ventriculography, Swan-Ganz measurements, and technetium-99m pyrophosphate imaging, the diagnostic accuracy of this electrocardiographic finding is about 83%. Importantly, this electrocardiographic finding is associated with a poor short-term prognosis with an in-hospital mortality rate of 31% versus 6% in patients without right ventricular involvement. This finding independently predicts short-term mortality and helps to rapidly risk-stratify patients with inferior myocardial infarction. Early recognition of this syndrome is important, because treatment often is considerably different from that in the usual inferior myocardial infarction. The classic clinical picture is a patient with an inferior infarction with hypotension, clear lungs, and elevated neck veins. These patients may become profoundly hypotensive to therapies that reduce preload, such as nitroglycerin therapy, which should be avoided in this situation. The combination of an infarcted, dilated right ventricle with pericardial restraint and ventricular interdependence results in diminished filling of the left ventricle and reduction in stroke volume, cardiac output, and blood pressure. The classic hemodynamic findings include a right atrial pressure/pulmonary capillary wedge pressure more than or equal to 0.8. These patients should be treated by maintenance of preload with fluid resuscitation. Although intravenous volume may resolve the hypotension, it also may lead to further right ventricular dilatation resulting in impingement via septal bulging on left ventricular filling. Dobutamine should then be considered to increase right ventricular contractility. In patients with significant left ventricular dysfunction and elevated pulmonary capillary wedge pressures, intra-aortic balloon pump support may be lifesaving. In addition to hemodynamic support, thrombolytic therapy should be at the forefront of therapy because there is a reduced incidence of right ventricular infarction in myocardial infarction with successful thrombolysis. Although the hemodynamic abnormalities in these patients often improve in 48 hours, patients with right ventricular infarction are more likely to develop high-grade atrioventricular block and require short- and long-term pacing.

CONCLUSIONS

Over the last 3 decades, the focus of the management of patients with acute myocardial infarction has dramatically changed. The initial life-saving therapies and technologies focused on electrical monitoring and electrical cardioversion for fatal ventricular arrhythmias that occurred with acute myocardial infarction. Over the past 10 years, large trials have refocused our efforts to limit infarct size, decrease congestive heart failure, and reduce recurrent ischemic events. These therapies include reperfusion with thrombolytic agents and primary angioplasty, use of aspirin, β-blockers, and ACE inhibitors. To maximize the benefits of these therapies, the house officer must recognize rapidly which patients are candidates for each of these therapies. Finally, the critically ill patient with cardiogenic shock, mechanical complications, or right ventricular infarction must be managed with the greatest expertise to reduce the high mortality associated with these disorders.

7

An Approach to the Long-Term Care of the Chronically Ill Child

Patricia M. Quigley edited by John J. Downes

Chronically ill children and their families face many crises together, beginning at the turbulent time of the child's initial diagnosis and acute illness. Once the acute severe episode resolves, many children with chronic disorders will benefit from care in a subacute hospital that focuses on ways to maximize the child's growth, overall development, and quality of life. This is accomplished by considering the complete child, including the interplay of medical, psychological, familial, and social factors. Often, children with chronic illness confront many issues that compound each other, making effective treatment difficult. By taking into account these interacting factors and needs, physicians, nurses, and other team members can devise a plan that will help the child reach his or her full potential. The plan of care should include management of the child's specific medical problems, as well as general aspects of care, including the child's nutritional state, physical rehabilitation requirements, psychological needs, family issues and support, and barriers to discharge. The plan of care should be geared toward safe discharge to the home and community with a cooperating primary care physician, preferably a general pediatrician, to oversee ongoing rehabilitation and developmental therapy and pediatric subspecialty care.

PATIENT SELECTION

Rapid medical advances in the care of critically ill infants and children, particularly the strides made in neonatology and neonatal surgery, have resulted in a growing number of children who have survived their initial insult but have developed chronic illness, often requiring special technical support for survival. Palfrey et al., estimated that, in 1990, the number of children in the United States who were technologically dependent was 101,800 with an overall prevalence rate of 0.16%. In comparing incident rates between 1987 and 1990, the fastest growing segments of this population were infants in the first year of life. There was a 36% increase in children requiring gastrostomy tubes and a 29% increase in those who were oxygen dependent. Care of these children can be costly. However, care in a subacute hospital is less expensive than in an acute care hospital, and home care is even less expensive.

In Maryland in 1987, for a child with a tracheostomy and supplemental oxygen with no ventilatory assistance, the estimated monthly cost in an acute care hospital ranged from $30,000 to $36,500; in a long-term care hospital the cost was $12,000; and home care cost was $5,300. Data from Pennsylvania (1994) reveals acute pediatric intensive care unit actual costs (not charges) averaged $49,260 per month. Costs in a respiratory rehabilitation unit averaged $33,000 monthly for a child requiring a tracheostomy and assisted ventilation. In the mid-1990s, the cost per month averaged $23,000 for the home care of infants and children needing a tracheostomy, mechanical ventilation, and 16 hours per day of nursing care. In addition to the monetary savings, a long-term hospital or home provides many other benefits to a chronically ill child, especially increased emphasis on the overall well-being of the child in a less hectic environment as opposed to the acute crisis management approach of an intensive care unit.

Appropriate candidates for hospitalization in a subacute or rehabilitation hospital include children with a chronic illness that requires definitive physical rehabilitation, developmental therapies, family training in care, and further medical care of the chronic illness. Every such hospital should have policies regarding the degree of acuity and stability a patient must achieve to be cared for by that institution. Of particular importance is the medical and technical support needed, as well as the daily number of nursing hours required for care. The level of care provided by a subacute hospital and the scope of services offered to the patients and families vary from institution to institution. For the child whose condition is terminal, a subacute facility may be an alternative to a hospice in providing palliative care, particularly if home hospice care is not desired by the family or care is deemed too complex for a traditional hospice program.

PRINCIPLES OF MEDICAL CARE

Children with a severe chronic illness invariably have multiple medical problems, and inadequate management of one problem can exacerbate others, making overall treatment difficult. For example, pain caused by decubital ulcers in a child with neuromuscular disease can lead to depression, causing anorexia and malnutrition, leading to worsening neuromuscular disease and poor wound healing. Also, certain medications or treatments used to treat one condition may adversely effect another. For instance, chest physiotherapy for atelectasis in a child with osteoporosis may lead to rib fractures unless it is done with a low-impact vibrator or similar device. Therefore, care of a chronically ill child on a long-term basis requires meticulous attention to detail while also considering the whole child and family.

Management of a child's condition in a subacute setting differs from that in an acute care facility. The goal over the long term is to provide effective therapy that enhances growth and development, minimizes pain, avoids adverse long-term effects, and fits into a schedule allowing for sleep, play, and therapeutic activities. The regimen and schedule also must be adapted for a home care setting when the child's discharge to home will occur soon.

Medications used in the acute care setting often must be changed for long-term care to minimize eventual side effects. For instance, furosemide provides a brisk diuresis needed during acute care, but has many potential long-term side effects such as diffuse nephrolithiasis, electrolyte imbalance, and hearing loss. Therefore, chronic diuretic management with chlorothiazide, which has slower onset of action and fewer complications, is preferable. The route of drug delivery varies in long-term care. In an acute care facility, a child often receives medications intravenously, whereas in chronic care the intravenous route rarely is needed unless the patient is acutely ill, or no other treatment options are available. Invasive procedures, including blood drawing, should be kept to a minimum. Attempts should be made to cluster painful procedures and provide prophylactic analgesia or sedation (e.g., enteral narcotics or benzodiazepines) to minimize physical and emotional trauma to the child. For children requiring regular use of intravenous medications for a prolonged period, an indwelling central venous line should be used. The timing of the child's medication and treatment regimen should be adjusted to permit adequate sleep and quiet rest. Most chronic medications and therapies can be grouped together and given mainly during waking hours.

NUTRITIONAL CONSIDERATIONS

Appropriate nutrition is essential in children with chronic illness. Many chronic conditions cause increased energy expenditure and/or malabsorption, causing normal caloric intake or balance of components to be inadequate. Children recovering from a severe acute illness or surgery, in whom energy demand increases and caloric intake decreases, are especially vulnerable to malnutrition.

In the child with chronic lung disease, inadequate caloric intake will lead to generalized weakness, thoracic pump failure, hypoventilation, failure to grow, and chronic respiratory failure. Malnutrition also can lead to decreased immune function, poor wound healing, and impaired ability to learn and function. Infants with bronchopulmonary dysplasia (BPD) frequently demonstrate this sequence of events. These infants often have an increased respiratory rate and work of breathing, and thus a high caloric requirement. Gastroesophageal reflux, emesis, and other feeding difficulties coupled with a propensity for interstitial pulmonary edema with increased fluid intake make it very difficult for the infants to take in enough calories to grow. Often they require a high caloric density formula as well as chronic diuretics to prevent edema. Infants with BPD need to maintain normal oxygenation at all times to grow and also to prevent pulmonary arterial hypertension. Moyer-Mileur et al., found that in infants with BPD who had pulse oximetry levels greater than 92% when awake may develop lower saturation levels during sleep. Infants with pulse oximetry levels of 88 to 91% during sleep grew at a rate of only 6.1 g/day, whereas those with levels greater than 92% grew at a rate of 17.3 g/day. Adequate body growth, especially height, is crucial for these infants and young children to promote lung growth and remodeling and facilitate recovery from BPD. In normal infants, alveolar replication from 50 million to approximately 300 million occurs mostly in the first 2 years and approaches the adult number by 8 years. Clinical experience with infants with chronic lung disease indicates much of this growth potential persists despite severe early injury; with linear growth at or above average velocity, new, effective lung tissue develops resulting in improved ventilation and eventual removal from mechanically assisted ventilation. Thus, growth is the key to recovery in these infants and children.

In children with neuromuscular disease, and those with progressively debilitating diseases such as AIDS, muscles weaken over time. However, their energy expenditure may increase as a result of increased work of breathing and intermittent hypoxia; concomitantly their ability to feed themselves and safely swallow may decline. Those caring for these children should be vigilant in watching for signs of cyanosis, weight loss, dysfunctional swallowing, and tracheal aspiration.

Long-term management of chronically ill children, particularly those with chronic lung disease and neuromuscular disease, should include a consultation and regular follow-up with a nutritionist. All of these children will have increased caloric needs and should be taught how to achieve an adequate intake. They should be monitored closely to ensure appropriate caloric intake and velocity of gains in weight and height. In infants with impaired growth, a high-calorie formula should be given; in older children, calorie supplements should be given. In those too debilitated to take in adequate calories, nasogastric tube or gastrostomy feedings will be necessary. In children with moderate to severe lung disease as a result of cystic fibrosis, nighttime gastrostomy feedings increase their weight, halt the decline of their lung function, increase their ability to perform activities of daily living, and increase their survival. This therapy also applies to adolescents or adults with progressive muscular dystrophy, respiratory failure, and early oral motor dysfunction.

REHABILITATION THERAPY

Infants and children with chronic illness are particularly vulnerable to developmental delay and functional deficits. With rehabilitation therapy, they usually can achieve significant improvement in physical and other developmental functions. These children will especially benefit from rehabilitation services during recovery from acute illness or surgery when they are prone to debilitation and developmental setbacks. Often, they will need ongoing services, particularly former preterm infants, those with major anomalies, and children with developmental delay or chronic muscle weakness.

Children who are born prematurely and those with multiple hospitalizations are at increased risk for developmental delay and should have their development monitored at regular intervals, e.g., every 6 to 12 months. Rehabilitation services include physical, occupational, speech and oral motor therapy, child life activities, and adaptive equipment services. A pediatric developmental specialist often can assist by monitoring a patient's developmental progress. Psychologic or neuropsychologic evaluations help monitor cognitive development and aid in devising strategies for cognitive deficits or learning disabilities.

Children with chronic lung disease with either chronic muscle weakness or acute weakness from disuse atrophy or debilitation, will benefit greatly from rehabilitation therapy. The goal of therapy is to improve respiratory mechanics and endurance. During therapy, children should be assessed for muscle weakness and muscle shortening, and an individualized program should be developed to strengthen weakened muscles and stretch shortened ones thus improving ventilatory efficiency. Any rehabilitation program for a child with chronic lung disease should be closely supervised by a therapist who is well trained in recognizing and responding to the signs and symptoms of respiratory distress and hypoxia. These children should receive heart and respiratory rate monitoring along with pulse oximetry during exercise. Endurance is enhanced by using progressively increased resistive loads. The muscle groups that require therapy are those of the shoulder girdle, thoracic cage, spine, abdomen, and diaphragm. Diaphragm strengthening is especially important because the diaphragm accounts for most of the work done during quiet breathing. Training the child to emphasize diaphragmatic breathing can decrease the use of respiratory accessory muscles and thus reduce energy expenditure. Relaxation exercises also may help train the child to keep accessory muscles relaxed. Corrected positioning and posture also can improve the mechanics of breathing. Children who have a tendency to develop atelectasis or pneumonia and have difficulty mobilizing their secretions should be taught techniques of deep breathing and forceful coughing. Anxiety can cause tightened muscles and rapid, shallow breathing that wastes energy; training and counseling should focus on minimizing the child's and parent's anxiety.

Supervised graded exercise can increase the ill child's level of fitness and possibly slow the progression of the disease. In children with asthma, regular aerobic exercise, such as jogging, improves multiple objective measures of exercise capabilities, including work capacity, oxygen consumption (a measure of fitness), and distance achieved. Also, the incidence of exercise-induced bronchospasm may decrease in a more fit individual because their minute ventilation, a stimulus for exercise-induced bronchospasm, decreases for a given level of work. In children with cystic fibrosis, exercise does not necessarily achieve an improvement in pulmonary function, but does increase the child's level of fitness and endurance. In children with neuromuscular disease, exercise testing can be used as a measure of progression of disease. Carefully graded exercises can improve the level of fitness in those with cerebral palsy and those with nonprogressive neuromuscular disease. In children with Duchenne muscular dystrophy, regular exercise may slow progression of muscle weakness. In addition to the objective measures of improvement with exercise, regular exercise and improved fitness also can improve patients' quality of life by increasing their dexterity and coordination, increasing their ability to participate in activities, and improving their overall sense of well-being.

In summary, rehabilitation services provide a myriad of benefits to the vulnerable child, including acceleration of development gains, improvement in endurance and muscle strength, increased range of extremity and trunk motion, prevention of contractures, and enhanced ability to perform activities of daily living. Such services usually should be provided in the acute hospital, the subacute institution, and for months or years at home and in school.

TRACHEOSTOMIES

Advances in the care of critically ill infants and children has led to the survival of many more children who require a long-term tracheostomy. Tracheostomies are needed in children with airway anomalies, craniofacial defects, and prolonged chronic respiratory failure requiring mechanical ventilation. Infants born prematurely have an increased incidence of airway anomalies, particularly subglottic stenosis. Once the child has recovered from the tracheostomy procedure, has safely undergone at least one tracheostomy tube change, and is medically stable, he or she can be transferred to a subacute hospital where rehabilitation to facilitate growth and development and the process involved in transitioning to home can begin.

The tracheostomy-related mortality rates for children with long-term tracheostomy beyond the perioperative period is about 2 to 4%. However, children with severe upper airway obstruction are at a much higher risk and are specifically at risk for death from accidental decannulation or tracheal tube obstruction. Children with tracheostomies require close supervision by a caregiver who is well-trained in care for patients with this condition. The caregiver must be proficient in cardiopulmonary resuscitation, suctioning, and changing of the tracheostomy tube, especially in emergency situations. They also must be able to recognize the symptoms of airway obstruction and indications for suctioning or changing of the tracheostomy tube. Children with tracheostomies also should be monitored with a cardiopulmonary monitor or pulse oximeter at all times when asleep or unattended, with a trained caregiver available to respond to their monitor. When outside the home or institution, caregivers should carry with them emergency supplies, including a suctioning device, tracheostomy tubes (correct size and one size smaller), tracheostomy strings, scissors, and a self-inflating bag/valve manual ventilation device (e.g., Ambu-bag). Before the child with a tracheostomy is discharged to home, all the caregivers need to receive intensive training regarding airway care and resuscitation with performance criteria to be passed before the child is discharged.

Children with long-term tracheostomies often have delay in language acquisition and expressive language skills, with particular problems with vowel production. These children have soft voices and poor articulation. They must have adequate airflow around their tracheostomy tube and up through the larynx to allow for speech. This can be achieved by using an uncuffed tracheostomy tube (or one in which the cuff is deflated) with an outer diameter approximately 75% of that of the tracheal lumen. Use of a speaking valve in older patients with a tracheostomy may aid in making speech louder and more clear but cannot be readily used with positive pressure ventilation. These valves are contraindicated in small infants and in patients with cuffed tracheostomy tubes or upper airway obstruction. The initial use of a speaking valve should be monitored carefully. Children learning to speak while on a ventilator must learn to speak on inhalation and later learn to adapt to speech on exhalation when they are weaned from the ventilator. A child with a tracheostomy may benefit from learning to communicate with sign language, which can be taught readily until vocal language skills can be mastered.

Children with tracheostomies are at increased risk for intrapulmonary aspiration caused by laryngeal incompetence. If aspiration is suspected, the child should undergo a radiographic study of his or her swallowing function. This can be assessed initially by putting methylene blue dye in the child's formula and noting the presence or absence of dye in the tracheal secretions. However, a formal swallowing evaluation will provide more detailed and useful information, especially if various consistencies of the oral material are offered during the study.

Often, children with tracheostomies will have difficulty enrolling in ordinary schools, because of the school administrator's fear of liability, financial concerns, insufficiently trained school staff, and staff anxiety. These children are protected by law, as are other disabled children, and should have no legal barriers to attending school. Health care workers educating school personnel is vital in eliminating fears of school staff and in providing the child with a safe school environment. For some children, especially those needing mechanical ventilation, a nurse or highly skilled personal attendant will be required.

PSYCHOSOCIAL ISSUES

It can be enormously stressful for the child and family to deal with the reality of chronic illness. The child faces being in some way "different" from his or her peers, which is especially difficult during adolescence when conforming to a peer group becomes paramount. Adolescents struggling to gain autonomy may become noncompliant with their treatment plan. They also may begin to grapple with issues of death and dying. Many children will have outward signs of their illness such as technological dependence, physical disabilities or limitations, or a wasted appearance. This may lead to a poor body image as well as a feeling of being stigmatized by society.

Children with chronic illness during the early stages of development may have difficulty developing a sense of trust and can have difficulty in developing feelings of competency. Young children in particular may feel guilty about having the disease, and older children may feel guilty about the burdens the disease places on the family. Almost 40% of children with chronic illness will have significant problems in school because of frequent absences, limited peer relationships, and learning difficulties.

Families experience tremendous stress when dealing with the impact of chronic illness. Parents often encounter expenses for treatment, equipment, and medications that are not covered by health insurance, which can place financial strains on the family. Parents often need time off from work because of their child's acute illness or hospitalization or to bring their child to a physician for follow-up care. The follow-up care of children with complicated medical needs may require visits to many specialists on a regular basis. For parents, time away from work may lead to difficulty in keeping a job.

Acute hospitalizations can be very disruptive and stressful for even the most seasoned parent of a chronically ill child and may force them to deal with the issues regarding the child's ultimate prognosis. Transfer from an acute care hospital to a subacute hospital also may be difficult for patients and their families. They must leave health care providers whom they have come to know and trust and form relationships with a new group of caregivers. Also, they must adjust to the less intensive style of a subacute hospital.

Parents of a child with chronic illness may feel a loss of control over their lives. For parents whose child requires nurses in the home, many find the lack of privacy in the home stressful. Parents also worry about the fate of their ill child when they are no longer able to care for them. Siblings also are affected because they receive less time and attention than their ill sibling, which can result in behavioral problems.

For these reasons, and many more, children with chronic illness and their families need an adequate support system and often benefit from professional counseling. These issues should be addressed with parents regularly, because parents may be reluctant to broach the subject to a physician or nurse, yet usually are relieved to talk about them once they are invited to open the dialogue. Concerns regarding the patient's prognosis and, if appropriate, specifics about death and dying should be addressed early because it is much easier than during a time of crisis.

Parents should be involved whenever possible in decisions regarding major changes in care, especially those affecting the child's prognosis. When sufficiently mature, a child should be included in discussions regarding care and prognosis. The child's opinion should be highly valued, particularly regarding the present quality of life and any end of life decisions. The patient's principal physicians should initiate all the major treatment changes or end of life discussions; these physicians likely are the most stable source of care for the child and have built up a level of trust with the family. For the chronically ill child, the principal physicians may consist of a combination of primary care physicians and subspecialists who have worked closely with the patient and family.

ICU Care for Adults with Chronic Illness

Rebecca D. Elon, Mary Jo Fishburn

ICU CARE FOR PATIENTS WITH CHRONIC ILLNESS

General Issues

When catastrophic events and life-threatening illness necessitate admission to the intensive care unit, the practitioner is most concerned with stabilizing the patient's vital functions. This requires an organ system approach analyzing cardiac, pulmonary, renal, endocrine, gastrointestinal, and nervous system parameters. The house officer, however, needs to view the intensive care unit admission as only one part of the patient's journey through the health care system. Typically, there is a history, often extensive for adults with chronic illness, and subsequent stages of recovery that may occur at home or in a postacute care setting. In a busy teaching hospital ICU, this may be overlooked as the present acute illness demands all of the physician's attention.

Teaching hospital ICUs often have "intensivists," or cardiologists or pulmonologists, who serve as unit attending physicians. The house officer should remember to identify the primary care physician who has worked with the patient over time. Communication is necessary for several reasons:

1. Important details of the history and response to therapy may be gleaned only through the primary care physician's understanding of the patient.

2. Important information regarding advance directives (that could have a great impact on ICU care) may be obtained from the primary care physician.
3. The primary care physician is typically the person responsible for the care after discharge from the ICU, making communication essential for continuity of care.
4. The primary care physician is often the one to whom families and patients turn for counseling and advice when making important decisions about their health care.

The trust and longitudinal doctor–patient relationship can be an important aspect of ICU care, even when the primary care physician is not the attending physician of record during the ICU stay.

Most patients admitted to the ICU will not have executed living wills or assigned a Durable Power of Attorney (DPOA) for health care decision making. It is necessary, though often awkward, to discuss advance directives once a critically ill patient has been admitted to the ICU. Often, this must be done with family of the patient if the patient is cognitively incapacitated acutely or chronically. In the absence of a DPOA or living will documents, written evidence of the patient's stated treatment preferences may be found in the outpatient medical record. Some states recognize documentation by physicians of such conversations in the medical record as a valid form of advance directives.

Understanding the patient's premorbid level of functioning is important for the ICU house officer. Even the most robust, vigorous, and active person with a serious illness requiring ICU care often becomes totally dependent in activities of daily living during the acute illness (Table 8.1). ICU patients often require assistance for bathing, grooming, bowel and bladder function and may need enteral tube feedings or parenteral nutrition. The most fundamental aspect of mobility, re-adjusting one's position in bed, often is lost during the acute illness. How fully and quickly the patient recovers functional capabilities after an acute or catastrophic illness may depend on the premorbid functional status. Appropriate planning for postacute care, whether it be discharge to home, to a rehabilitation center, to subacute facility, nursing home, or assisted living setting, will largely depend on the pa-

Table 8.1
Levels of Functional Capability

Activities of daily living (ADL)
(Basic human functions. Ability to perform independently may be impaired by chronic or acute illness)
- Bathing
- Dressing
- Grooming
- Toileting
- Ambulating / Transferring
- Feeding

Instrumental activities of daily living (IADL)
(Higher level functions for independent living. Adults either do these themselves, have a family member perform the task, or hire outside help to accomplish IADLs)
- Driving a car or using public transportation
- Personal finances
- Shopping
- Cooking
- Cleaning
- Laundry
- Using telephone

Social functioning
- Family role
- Occupational role
- Avocations
- Emotional
- Spiritual

tient's functional status and potential for independent living in the future. Functional derangements of organ systems (such as heart failure, respiratory failure, renal failure) are typically the rationale for ICU care. Functional deficits of the patient, however, are the rationale for most long-term care or chronic care services.

Approach to Older Patients in the ICU

Advanced age and preexisting cognitive impairment predispose older patients to delirium during their ICU admission. A prospective study of delirium in elderly patients admitted to general medical and surgical units in a teaching hospital found that 11% were delirious at the time of admission. An additional 31% developed new onset delirium during the hospitalization, and 34% developed individual symptoms of delirium without meeting full criteria. This rate of 76% of elderly developing signs and symptoms of cognitive dysfunction during hospitalization is of concern. The percentage of potentially avoidable delirium is uncertain, although adverse reaction to drugs constitutes one category the ICU physician should attempt to minimize. Drugs that may cause delirium in older patients include sedative/hypnotics, H_2 antagonists, narcotics, anticholinergics, centrally acting antihypertensives, antiparkinsonians, lidocaine, and drugs such as diuretics that may cause metabolic derangements. Alcohol or benzodiazepine withdrawal also may cause delirium.

Although delirium typically is triggered by an acute illness, metabolic derangement, intoxication, or drug side effect and is potentially reversible, one prospective study found that only 4% of delirious hospitalized elderly had resolution of all cognitive symptoms before discharge. At 3 months, 21% were back to baseline, and at 6 months, an additional 18% had regained their cognitive functions. This leaves 57% of patients with hospital-associated delirium remaining cognitively impaired 6 months after the acute event. Further studies into the pathophysiology of delirium are needed before implementing targeted prevention strategies.

Simple strategies, such as avoiding sensory overload and sensory deprivation; maximizing frequent human contact including liberal family visitation; limiting use of restraints and psychotropic drugs; and avoiding polypharmacy, may help decrease the rate of delirium (Table 8.2). Interventional trials, however, are lacking.

The proportion of elderly patients admitted to ICUs is higher in the USA than in other countries (Table 8.3). Although Japan has a higher percentage of elderly people than the USA, the percentage receiving ICU care is much lower. This could mean that older Japanese are healthier or younger Japanese are sicker. Alternatively, it could mean that Japanese physicians exclude more elderly people from ICU care than their American counterparts.

Although unadjusted mortality data indicate a higher rate of death for elderly ICU patients (Table 8.4), studies controlling for severity of illness indicate that age is a less important predictor than physiologic derangement. Three commonly used prognostic scoring systems (Acute Physiology and Chronic Health Evalu-

Table 8.2
Interventions to Minimize Risk of Delirium

Avoid sensory overload
- Maintain normal day/night lighting/darkness patterns
- Place bed near window
- Have monitor and IV alarms alert nursing staff without disturbing patient
- Limit number of phlebotomies, injections, painful examinations
- Limit staff noise at night

Avoid sensory deprivation
- Obtain and use patient's personal equipment, such as hearing aides and eye glasses to promote communication
- Encourage family visits
- Encourage staff to communicate and orient patient frequently

Minimizes use of potentially psychoactive medication
- Proton pump inhibitors appear to have less CNS impact than H_2 blockers
- Anticholinergic drugs should be avoided when possible
- Avoid long-acting benzodiazepines
- Titrate pain medications to minimize side effect

Avoid restraints

Table 8.3
Elderly ICU Admits in USA vs. Other Countries

Country	ICU Admits > 65 Years Old (%)
USA	48
Wales	52
Canada	26
Japan	30
France	30
New Zealand	17

Table 8.4
Mortality After Intensive Care Depends More on Severity of Illness than Age

Age	Unadjusted Hospital Mortality for ICU Patients (%)*
45	12–15
46–64	12–27
⩾65	34–37
⩾85	38

*Severity of illness adjustment accounts for up to 85% of the variance between ages.

ation [APACHE III]; Mortality Prediction Model [MPM II]; and Simplified Acute Physiology Score [APS II]) use age as one of the variables to predict outcomes. The variance accounted for by age in these measures is small.

In one study, 90% of elderly patients admitted to the ICU were living independently before their illness, and 80% were living independently 1 year after ICU discharge. ICU stays of greater than 1 week decreased the percentage to 70% living independently at 1 year.

The Society of Critical Care Medicine ethics committee discourages admission of elderly individuals to the ICU with poor functional status because of irreversible, chronic illness. Patients with imminently fatal illness or permanent unconsciousness should not be placed in the ICU. It is rational, however, to admit elderly patients with potentially curable conditions to the ICU with the assumption that after a short therapeutic trial, therapy can be withdrawn if clinical status does not improve, and the diagnosis and prognosis indicate no hope for recovery. Age alone should not be the sole determinant in deciding whether or not to admit an acutely ill patient to the ICU.

A study of the cost of care of octogenarians, nonagenarians, and centenarians revealed that very old patients receive a lower intensity care, and are more likely to be cared for in nonteaching hospitals. For elderly patients dying during hospitalization, hospital costs were much higher than for those who survived. However, this difference declined with age. In the 60- to 69-year-old group, decedents cost per hospitalization was 141% higher than survivors. For those 100 years old and older, the cost was 23% higher. This difference is likely because older patients are offered less aggressive care on the basis of age, have advance directives limiting care, receive fewer surgical interventions, and are nursing facility residents discharged more quickly than community-dwelling elderly.

Rehabilitation Approach to the ICU Patient

Health care providers consider rehabilitation an "afterthought"; a process that begins after the acute care needs have been met. The best ICU care, however, includes a rehabilitation approach as part of its acute medical intervention. To achieve the optimal long-term rehabilitation outcomes, certain principles must be addressed during the acute treatment phase. Several strategies or concepts are central to this approach:

1. Prevention of injury
2. Reduction of pathology to a minimum
3. Prevention of secondary complications and disabilities (e.g., debility, decubiti, deep venous thrombosis, contractures)
4. Enhancement of the function of involved systems (e.g., through coma stimulation or communication augmentation)
5. Enhancement of the function of uninvolved systems
6. Development of systematic compensatory strategies (e.g., alternative communication techniques for those on a ventilator, alternative swallowing techniques, bowel program for neurogenic incontinence)

Sequelae of Bed Rest

Prolonged bed rest leads to several physiologic changes that adversely affect the whole person and prolongs institutionalization and/or dependence on others. One of the most significant musculoskeletal effects is disuse weakness. Ten to fifteen percent of muscle strength is lost per week of complete bed rest. After 3 to 5 weeks, an estimated 50% deficit in muscle strength may be seen. Some of the electron microscopic changes seen in muscle after 6 weeks of immobilization are fiber degeneration and an increased proportion of fat and fibrous tissue.

Weakness and atrophy begin with the gravity resistors, the musculature of the trunk and the lower extremities in particular. With time, generalized weakness and atrophy will occur. Physiologically, muscle changes include reduced oxidative enzyme activity, resulting in lowered tolerance to oxygen debt and earlier, longer accumulation of lactic acid. This leads to greater cardiovascular demand with muscle use. Increased catabolism is also seen, including muscle protein loss.

Another significant musculoskeletal consequence of prolonged bed rest is the development of contractures. A contracture, the lack of full passive range of motion because of soft-tissue shortening, can result from any one, or combination, of three anatomic limits: muscle, joint capsule, or other connective tissue. Myogenic and connective tissue contractures are most frequently associated with immobility.

Three factors contribute to the development of a contracture: limb position, duration of immobilization, and mobilization of unaffected parts. When the full range of motion is not maintained by activity, two-jointed muscles are usually the first to become shortened (hamstrings, back muscles, tensor fasciae latae, rectus femoris, and gastrocnemius are the most common). This is dictated by a tendency to assume a typical position of comfort: abduction of the lower limb with external rotation and flexion at the hip, flexion at the knee, and plantar flexion and inversion at the ankle. In this position, the patient will have risk for contracture at any joint in the lower extremity. In addition, this position promotes concurrent pressure over the fibular head, which increases the risk of peroneal nerve palsy and associated foot drop.

A contracture at any joint will reduce mobility and/or self-care capability. For example, hip flexion contractures reduce hip extension during gait, shorten stride, and promote increased lumbar lordosis. Hamstring muscles become relatively shorter, resulting in knee flexion tightness. These gait deviations result in an increase in energy expenditure during ambulation. Contractures of the upper limb may cause impairment of reaching, dressing, feeding, and fine motor tasks.

Degenerative joint disease and immobilization osteoporosis also have been associated with prolonged immobility. Animal studies have shown that immobility thickens and tightens the joint capsule and destroys cartilage. Increased trabecular bone resorption also occurs, with associated hypercalcemia (especially seen in children, young adults, and elderly patients with Paget's disease), hypercalciuria, and, ultimately, osteoporosis.

Immobility also adversely affects cardiovascular capacity. Four common manifestations of these effects are listed:

1. Redistribution of body fluids
2. Orthostatic hypotension
3. Cardiovascular deconditioning
4. Increased thromboembolic disease

Blood viscosity increases due to diuresis-induced reduction in plasma volume (inhibited antidiuretic hormone release) and increases the risk of deep venous thrombosis. Orthostatic hypotension can develop even after a few days of bed rest, because the normal compensatory response of vasoconstriction, increased heart rate, and blood pressure on assuming upright position become impaired. Patients with major trauma, including thermal as well as mechanical trauma, systemic disease, or advanced age, are especially prone to orthostatic hypotension.

Cardiovascular deconditioning is the result of reduced cardiac output, primarily through reduced stroke volume, over weeks of immobility. An estimated decline in end-diastolic ventricular volume of 6 to 11% can occur after 2 weeks of bed rest. In addition to these changes, the resting heart rate progressively increases. Exercise tolerance and work capacity become progressively impaired. Reduced skeletal muscle functional capacity adds to this decline. Decreased muscle strength and endurance, reduced pumping effect of lower extremity muscles, poor venous return, and overall decreased metabolic activity of muscle all contribute.

The respiratory consequences to prolonged immobility can be life threatening. Mechanical restriction of tidal volume, minute volume, and functional ventilatory reserve capacity occurs as a result of reduced diaphragmatic and intercostal movements during recumbency. Respiratory rate increases to compensate. The risk of atelectasis and pneumonia is increased because secretions tend to accumulate in dependent portions of the lung, and coughing is less effective in the supine position. Total lung-diffusing capacity and pulmonary blood flow volume decline. Ventilation–perfusion ratios change in dependent areas of the lungs, with poor ventilation and over perfusion, which reduces arterial oxygenation.

Numerous endocrine and metabolic changes also occur:

1. Increased catabolism with protein breakdown and increased nitrogen loss
2. Increased excretion of potassium, sodium, phosphorous, and calcium
3. Increased bone resorption in response to increased parathyroid hormone release

4. Reduced androgen hormones
5. Reduced adrenal responsiveness

Bladder function often is impaired in the bed-bound patient. Reduced intra-abdominal pressure in the supine position increases the risk of urinary retention and cystitis. Bladder stones (estimated to occur in 15 to 30% of immobilized patients) may form as a result of retention and hypercalciuria of immobility.

Common gastrointestinal sequelae of bed rest include bowel impaction as a result of reduced peristalsis. Nutritional decline is common in acutely ill patients as a result of anorexia, inability to eat, increased caloric demands from acute illness and delays in use of enteral or parenteral nutritional support by the medical or surgical team.

Adverse neurologic effects because of the sensory and psychosocial deprivation of bed rest can lead to confusion, disorientation, increased anxiety and/or depression, and reduced psychomotor skills and coordination.

Functionally, sustained bed rest leads to general debility or weakness, which can be severe enough to incapacitate the individual completely. Common consequences also include muscular pain, backaches, gait instability, and falls.

Interventions/Prevention. Early mobilization, such as daily out-of-bed-to-chair activity, for tolerated sitting times is the initial step to prevent the sequelae of bed rest. Avoid prescribing strict bed rest unless absolutely necessary, and allow bathroom privileges or use a bedside commode whenever possible. Encourage the patient to stand for 30 to 60 seconds whenever transferring from bed to chair. The nursing staff should be diligent in helping patients change position in bed to prevent decubiti and pulmonary complications. An air-fluid specialized bed may help to prevent skin breakdown or help staff respond to early signs of skin compromise.

Appropriate positioning of limbs while in bed with the use of pillows and/or splints, such as the derotation splint, can prevent contractures, decubiti, and the postural abnormalities that can result in subsequent pain and gait dysfunction.

Daily range of motion activity, either passively (through

nursing and/or therapists) or actively (through patient education and coaching), prevents contractures and deep venous thrombosis. Mild contractures improve with prolonged terminal passive stretch for 20 to 30 minutes twice daily. Severe collagenous contractures require heat as well as prolonged stretch for a similar period and schedule. If the contracture is muscular, serial casting or dynamic splinting for prolonged periods (days) may be required.

A bowel program, such as every other day suppository, can prevent impaction and more severe gastrointestinal conse-

Table 8.5
Guidelines for Remobilizing the Medically Complex Patient

1. Intervention for orthostatic hypotension
   a. Change position slowly and provide frequent rest periods with activity
   b. Provide mechanical support of blood pressure (improves venous return) with TED hose and abdominal binder
2. Cardiac precautions
   a. Monitor closely and stop activity for evidence of cardiac ischemia (systolic blood pressure drop with activity, symptoms such as profound fatigue, chest pain, dyspnea)
   b. Assess oxygen saturation with activity with pulse oximetry, and consider oxygen supplementation
   c. Avoid activity within 1 hour after meals if cardiac reserve is significantly limited, because the mesenteric blood flow demand after meals creates a physiologic decline in blood volume available for activity
   d. Treat severe anemia to promote optimal oxygen-carrying capacity of the blood
   e. Maximal heart rate should not exceed 70% of age-predicted maximum (220−age) in acute or subacute cardiac conditions, or 80% of 220−age if cardiac history suggests tendency toward cardiac compromise with activity (congestive heart failure, etc.)
3. Considerations with bleeding diatheses, such as anticoagulation or hemophilia
   a. Avoid vigorous heat
   b. Avoid stretch of tissue
4. Pulmonary precautions
   a. Assess if patient has oxygen desaturation with activity, or with sleep, using pulse oximetry, and supplement if O_2 saturations consistently drop below 88%
   b. Educate on pulmonary principles, such as pursed lip breathing and pulmonary hygiene
5. Special considerations for individuals with multiple sclerosis
   a. Do not over-fatigue
   b. Do not over-heat

quences such as small bowel obstruction. Adequate hydration is essential to prevent orthostatic hypotension and bowel and bladder sequelae. An upright posture during bowel and bladder elimination will promote more effective emptying.

Pulmonary hygiene, including incentive spirometry, deep breathing exercises, coughing, adequate hydration, and chest percussion will prevent retained secretions and atelectasis.

Intervention should be prescribed to prevent deep venous thrombosis, a common sequelae of prolonged immobility. If Sequential Compression Devices (SCDs) are used, the patient must wear it at all times when not exercising for it to be effective. Several medical alternatives, including heparin, warfarin, or low molecular weight heparin, should be considered. Education of the patient to perform ankle-pump exercises every 20 minutes can also be effective.

When prolonged immobilization is no longer necessary, cardiac reconditioning should begin with 65% maximal heart rate, advancing to 70 to 80% of maximal age-adjusted heart rate as activity tolerance improves. Maximal age-adjusted heart rate is estimated by the formula (220−age) (Table 8.5). A warm-up exercise program is essential to prevent undue stress on the heart. A cool-down exercise program will enhance venous return, prevent post exercise hypotension, provide better elimination of lactic acid, and induce release of exercise-related catecholamine and heat.

Suggested Reading

DeLateur BJ. The spectrum of physical treatment. In: Hays RM, Stolov WC, Kraft GH, eds. The management of chronic disease and disability: basic principles. New York: Demos, 1994.

Fein AM, Adelman RD. Critical illness in the elderly. Clin Geriatr Med 1994;10:1–237.

9

Cardiac Surgery Intensive Care

Jeff Dodd-o, Daniel Nyhan

When admitting a patient to the cardiac surgical intensive care unit, the most important assessment is for the airway. The patient without a secure airway will not ventilate and oxygenate well. With a compromised myocardium, elevated carbon dioxide and diminished oxygen can lead to worsening myocardial ischemia. The most conservative approach for treatment is to maintain the airway artificially. The process of extubating the patient, either postoperatively or after semielective intubation, is associated with cardiovascular stresses. Endotracheal extubation should be performed maintaining optimal hemodynamics and sometimes requires beta blockade to minimize the stress to the injured myocardium. Whether to extubate and the timing and management of extubation have to be individualized to the patient's condition. Maintenance on a ventilator can assure oxygenation and carbon dioxide removal and is often the most conservative approach to treatment after cardiac surgery.

POSTOPERATIVE MANAGEMENT OF PATIENTS AFTER CARDIAC SURGERY

The objectives in the immediate postoperative period (0 to 8 hours) include the following:

1. Optimize hemodynamics
2. Maintain gas exchange and wean from mechanical ventilation

3. Establish normothermia
4. Optimize fluid and electrolyte balance
5. Monitor blood loss, correct coagulopathy, and treat if necessary
6. Optimize emergence from anesthesia/pain management and neuromuscular function (reverse neuromuscular blockers, if necessary) and treat shivering.

The objectives 8 or 12 to 48 hours postoperatively include the following:

1. Nervous system: full neurologic assessment and pain management
2. Cardiovascular: continued weaning/removal of cardiovascular support (pharmacologic and/or mechanical), prophylaxis/treatment of Dysrhythmias (particularly atrial fibrillation/flutter)
3. Pulmonary: optimization of gas exchange and ventilation (pulmonary toilet) postextubation and removal of chest tubes
4. Fluid/electrolytes: removal of intravascular and total body fluid overload through diuresis. Monitoring/repletion of electrolytes
5. Transfer to subacute setting

DETAILED SYSTEM EVALUATION

Neurologic

Neurological complications are common after cardiac surgery. Focal deficits may be found in up to 6% of patients (CAB ~ 3%, valves < 2%, combined CAB and valves ~ 6%) and may be severe in 2% of patients. More refined and sensitive tests of fine motor function, psychological function, etc., demonstrate decrements in 30 to 50% of patients. The incidence of these complications may increase if the risk factors increase in the population having surgery (as in older patients, emergency surgery, poor left ventricular function, associated peripheral vascular disease). Neurological deficits may occur intraoperatively, but a large percentage occurs postoperatively after a period during which the patient was neurologically intact. The etiology of postoperative neurological deficits is multifactorial (embolic, hypoperfusion, hemorrhagic, metabolic), but onset in the postoperative period may reflect the importance of optimizing hemodynamics, temperature, and glucose homeostasis postoperatively.

Altered Mental Status: Nonfocal

Etiologies Etiologies of nonfocal altered mental status include: metabolic, infectious, neoplastic, traumatic, and drug factors.

Metabolic Changes in mental status can be caused by: hypoxemia, hypercarbia, acidosis, hypo/hypernatremia, hypo/hyperglycemia, hypercalcemia, hypermagnesemia, hyperphosphatemia, elevated ammonia, and uremia ("restless legs," areflexia, and distal sensory loss). Deficiencies of thiamine, vitamin B12, and niacin are other causes. Hyper/hypoadrenalism are less common, the latter usually associated with hypotension). Hypothyroidism, Myasthenia Gravis, Amyloid or Guillain-Barré may also exhibit nonfocal neurological features.

Infectious Although the incidence of CSF infection is low in patients who have not had neuraxial analgesia or a spinal drain unless they are otherwise immunocompromised (e.g., HIV, asplenic, dialysis, absolute neutrophil count < 1000, Cushing), sepsis (not directly involving the CSF) can cause mental status changes.

Neoplasm Mass effects of neoplasm can be acutely exacerbated by bleeding while the patient is anticoagulated for bypass.

Cerebrovascular The most common etiology of acute deterioration in the cardiac surgery population is stroke secondary to thrombosis, hemorrhage, or hypoperfusion. Although a stroke frequently presents as a unilateral functional deficit, there may not be focal features. Moreover, the location of stroke may make focal features less obvious (e.g., occipital stroke with visual deficit).

Drugs/Drug Withdrawal This factor is a result of either the exposure to new agents or the withdrawal from agents (e.g., alcohol, "asleep" medications) that the patient was taking previously.

Focal Neurological Deficits

It is useful to discuss these events in three ways: 1) completeness, 2) anatomical distribution, and 3) etiology.

Transient ischemic attacks resolve in less than 24 hours if carotid disease is present, and less than 72 hours if the patient has posterior disease. If a neurological defect is stable in less than 24 hours (carotid disease) or less than 72 hours (posterior disease) the clinical defect is "a stroke in evolution." A completed stroke indicates that the deficit exists, but the patient is stable more than 24 hours (carotid disease) or more than 72 hours (posterior disease). When the patient has unilateral signs, the anterior circulation is involved. The term "watershed" refers to the area of the brain that is on the border of the region perfused by either the anterior or posterior circulations and may be especially vulnerable to hypoperfusion.

The etiology of neurological injury in the cardiac surgery patient is embolic in the majority of patients. Cannulation and perfusion of an atherosclerotic aorta is the most frequent cause of emboli. However, gaseous emboli (in a true open heart), vegetations on cardiac valves, and thrombus formation in the setting of atrial fibrillation or myocardial infarction are other sources of emboli in these patients. As in any patient, cerebrovascular disease may be a source of emboli; however, cerebral hypoperfusion (without emboli) may be caused by neurological insults. The alterations in pressure and flow patterns on CPB may have even greater effects on cerebral perfusion in patients with disease of cerebral vessels and in patients who have cerebrovascular autoregulation modulated by CPB itself. Finally, intracerebral hemorrhage, though not common, may occur with anticoagulation.

In the event of a **functional deficit,** serial physical examinations are performed to determine progression, stability or resolution of the deficit, and to rule out peripheral nerve involvement. CT or MRI scans distinguish hemorrhagic from nonhemorrhagic events and define the extent of tissue involvement. A cardiac ECHO should be performed to rule out a cardiac source for emboli.

In patients who have had cardiac surgery, myopathies and polyneuropathies of new onset are rare in the early postoperative period. Mononeuropathies, such as upper-extremity weakness secondary to brachial plexus stretching, lower-extremity deficits secondary to nerve damage, vocal cord paralysis, phrenic nerve paralysis, and Horners syndrome, are complications in cardiac patients.

Management of patients with postoperative neurological injury includes the following:

1. Symptomatic care (e.g., occupational therapy, speech therapy, airway management, etc.)
2. Addressing the cause—treat atrial fibrillation (cardioversion and pharmacotherapy)
3. Anticoagulation (if not contraindicated) for atrial fibrillation

Cardiovascular

Ventricular Function

The principle goal is to assure adequate tissue perfusion to all parts of the body. Clinical indications of adequate tissue perfusion include warm extremities, peripheral pulses, and evidence of normal end-organ function (normal mentation, EKG without ischemia, good urine output). By contrast, indications of inadequate tissue perfusion include altered mental status, oliguria, hypotension, and acidosis. Because of the central responsibility of the heart in organ perfusion, it is important to rule out inadequate myocardial performance as a contributor when tissue hypoperfusion is suspected.

Low cardiac output and hypoperfusion is associated with an increased incidence of multi-organ failure and death. Patients may have poor left ventricular function preoperatively or it may develop acutely postoperatively during periods of stress/ischemia, tamponade, or valvular dysfunction. In patients with cardiogenic shock, the management depends on the cause and optimizing hemodynamics with fluids, inotropes, ventricular afterload reduction, and mechanical assistance (intra-aortic balloon pump). Pharmacologic agents used to treat low cardiac output include the following:

1. **Inotropes.** This type of agent includes dopamine (tends to cause tachycardia), dobutamine (tends to decrease SVR), epinephrine (low-dose decreases SVR, higher dose increases SVR and heart rate), and norepinephrine (increases SVR, no change or decrease in heart rate).
2. **Afterload reduction.** Nitrovasodilators, such as nitroprusside and nitroglycerin, are used, the latter if pulmonary vascular pressures are elevated disproportionally.

3. **Phosphodiesterase inhibitors.** Agents such as amrinone and milrinone are used, especially if pulmonary pressures are elevated.
4. **Converting-enzyme (ACE) inhibitors.** These are more suitable for chronic use because of inability to titrate acutely.
5. **Calcium antagonists.** These lower SVR and BP but their negative inotropic effect render these agents unsuitable if ventricular function is compromised. They should be used for postoperative hypertension (vide infra) or when myocardial ischemia is secondary to vasospasm of either grafts or native vessels (vide infra). Nicardipine is available intravenously.

Postoperative Hypertension Significant hypertension occurs frequently postoperatively in cardiac surgery patients. The etiology of this postoperative hypertension is multifactorial and includes the following:

1. Preoperative hypertension
2. Perioperative factors, such as shivering, pain, manipulation of the great intrathoracic vessels intraoperatively
3. Metabolic factors, such as hypoxia and hypercarbia

The complications of postoperative hypertension are myocardial ischemia as a result of an imbalance of myocardial oxygen supply and demand; hypertension-induced organ change, e.g., renal, cerebral; and disruption of surgical sites (graft anastomosis, aortotomy, cannulation sites, etc.).

Pharmacological agents used to treat postoperative hypertension include the following:

1. Sodium nitroprusside (this is the mainstay of treatment)
2. Hydralazine
3. Prazosin
4. Nifedipine (sublingually) or intravenous calcium antagonists (nicardipine)

Ventricular Dysrhythmias

Normal cardiac rhythm depends on the following:

1. The dominance of a single pacemaker (SA node)
2. The presence of a conduction system, which allows fast and

uniform conduction of action potential (atrial conduction system, AV node and bundle of His)

3. A long uniform duration of action potential (assured by Purkinje fiber action potential, which lasts even longer than that of the ventricular muscle fibers).

Normal myocyte membrane potential is maintained at baseline by the Na:K ATP pump to keep intracellular K high and intracellular Na low. The membrane depolarizes to a threshold potential at which point *Phase 0* begins. During *Phase 0,* potential-dependent fast Na channels open and Na enters the cell. Slow Na:Ca channels also allow entry of this cation. During the short duration of *Phase 1* (close fast Na channels) and *Phase 2* (decreasing slow Na:Ca entrance rate with stable K exit rate), there is a plateau. During *Phase 3* (little Na:Ca exit with stable/increasing K+ entrance), repolarization begins and is completed as potassium outflow from the cell occurs to a limited extent.

Antiarrhythmics are classified on the basis of their effect on the cardiac action potential. Their goal is to prolong the refractory period (as measured by the Q-T interval) and/or decrease the ability to conduct.

Class 1 agents are local anesthetics (block fast Na^+ channels) that depress myocardial SA node cell membranes by slowing *Phase 0* depolarization. They also depress conduction velocity and inhibit spontaneous diastolic depolarization (decrease Na entrance during *Phase 4* so cells maintain their intracellular negativity). The *1a* agents (Procainamide and Quinidine) depress *Phase 0* and significantly depress depolarization, prolong action potential duration and the effective refractory period (ERP). This is seen on EKG as prolonged QRS and QT, with risk of "Torsades des pointes." One does not get a prolonged PR interval because of the vagolytic effects of these agents (these agents actually shorten the PR interval). Other side effects include GI upset, Lupus-like reaction, and (rarely) hemolysis with agranulocytosis. Quinidine increases serum digoxin levels. The *1b* agents (lidocaine and phenytoin) depress *Phase 0* minimally and shorten ERP (shortened QT interval and, with phenytoin, shortened PR). These are effective mainly for ventricular (not atrial) dysrhythmias, particularly if as a result of ischemia (peri-MI). Phenytoin may increase availability of protein-bound compounds (e.g., warfarin). Phenytoin is used for treating digoxin toxicity and sometimes "Torsades des pointes." The *1c* agents significantly depress depolarization, slow conduction, prolong the action potential and ERP. Because of their effect on *Phase 0,* these agents have less efficacy at more negative resting potential (i.e., when driving force for Na entry is greater), such as hypokalemia. Conversely, under myocardial ischemia (when transmembrane potential is less), the efficacy of the *lc* agent is enhanced. Thus, they decrease the disparity in duration of action potentials in normal (shortens refractory period) and ischemic (prolongs refractory period) tissue, improving uniform spread of depolarization wave across the myocardium.

Class 2 (Propranolol) agents are antisympathetic, block *Phase 4* depolarization, slow conduction, prolong ERP and action potential.

Class 3 agents prolong all phases of action potential, prolong repolarization, slow conduction, and prolong ERP.

Class 4 agents block calcium channels, and are most effective with dysrhythmias involving AV and SA node.

Atrial Dysrhythmias

Clinically significant atrial arrhythmias (atrial fibrillation) occur in approximately 40% of postoperative cardiac patients. The manifestation of atrial arrhythmias is multifactorial:

1. Underlying disease
2. Intra-operative manipulation (cannulae, etc.)
3. Cardiac arrest period (during aortic cross clamping)
4. Electrolyte imbalance
5. Chamber distension
6. Acid-base disturbance, etc.

Atrial fibrillation may result in thrombus formation (and thus embolization), compromised hemodynamics (low blood pressure, or compromised organ perfusion) (decreased urine output, fluid retention, etc.). Management consists of the following:

1. Treat entities that may precipitate atrial fibrillation
2. Convert to sinus rhythm with cardioversion (if recent onset or anticoagulated)

3. Attempt to convert to sinus rhythm with pharmacotherapy (procainamide, amiodarone)
4. Control ventricular response with digoxin or diltiazem
5. Anticoagulate (heparin ± oral anticoagulants)

Ischemic EKG Changes in the Postoperative Cardiac Patient

ST- and T-wave changes are a frequent occurrence postoperatively. The physician must identify patients whose EKG changes result from causes that require immediate treatment (e.g., surgical revision of an anastomosis, angioplasty, pharmacological treatment of vasospasm in either native coronaries or in arterial conduits). The assessment of these patients requires an overall analysis of preoperative, intraoperative, and postoperative information including the following:

1. Comparison of pre-, intra-, and postoperative EKGs as well as a determination of whether the patient was actively ischemic (with or without EKG changes) before aortic cross-clamping constitutes important information
2. Determination of the location and extent of the patient's native coronary lesions, the surgeon's satisfaction with revascularization (i.e., size and flow in mammary graft, size of the coronary vessel, runoff, and potential for graft occlusion)
3. Correlation between EKG changes and location of coronary disease and efficacy of revascularization
4. Evaluation of ventricular function
5. Determination of whether the EKG changes occur in the setting of dysrhythmias

These patients represent a frequent diagnostic dilemma for the physician. However, a patient who develops acute onset ST elevation in a distribution whose revascularization was technically problematic; who concurrently has a decrement in regional wall motion in that territory (as demonstrated by TEE); and who has developed malignant arrhythmias represents an easy decision for the physician. Such a patient should go directly to the OR or to the Cath Lab. In contrast, a patient who has minimum ST change confined to a distribution where further augmentation of revascularization is not feasible and who has normal ventricular function without dysrhythmias is a patient that might require observation only. Many patients fall between these two extremes. The specific management of any patient depends on the experience and comfort level of the physician, as well as what evolves with the patient over time.

Pulmonary Vascular Disease

Background Abnormalities of the pulmonary circulation (elevated pulmonary vascular pressures and elevated pulmonary vascular resistance) represent a frequent problem in both adults and children who have had cardiac surgery. Increased pulmonary vascular pressures, which may or may not have progressed to the point of causing changes in pulmonary vascular resistance, are sometimes recognized preoperatively. Factors that predispose to disturbances in pulmonary vasoregulation include the following:

1. Primary pulmonary hypertension
2. Secondary pulmonary hypertension, associated with mitral valve disease, left ventricular failure, COPD, and congenital heart disease
3. Cardiopulmonary bypass
4. Drugs (e.g., protamine-acutely)
5. Mechanical (increased intrathoracic pressures)

Clinical Manifestations Abnormalities of the pulmonary circulation manifest themselves by the following:

1. Increased pulmonary vascular pressures
2. Increased pulmonary vascular pressures and increased pulmonary vascular resistance
3. Right ventricular changes, such as failure (increased CVP, hepar, pedal edema, etc.)
4. Right ventricular ischemia (secondary to decreased right coronary perfusion pressure)
5. Dysrhythmias (atrial and ventricular)

Physiology of the Pulmonary Circulation/Interpretation of Pulmonary Hemodynamics The diagnosis of abnormalities in pulmonary vascular pressures with or without increases in pulmonary vascular resistance is contingent upon an accurate measurement of flow (i.e., cardiac output) and a concomitant accurate measurement of the pulmonary vascular pressure gradient (i.e., the upstream or driving pulmonary pressure minus the downstream pressure). Cardiac output is measured using the thermodilution cardiac output technique, and the pulmonary vascular pressures are measured using an appropriately positioned Swan-Ganz catheter. The pulmonary artery occlusion pressure is used to indicate downstream pressure. It is critically important to distinguish elevations in pulmonary vascular pressure with and without changes in pulmonary vascular resistance. This distinction not only has prognostic implications, but also has potential therapeutic implications. For example, elevated pulmonary vascular pressures that result passively from an increase in downstream pressures can be treated effectively by measures aimed at augmenting left ventricular output (i.e., inotropes and left ventricular afterload reduction). In contrast, elevations in pulmonary vascular pressures resulting from disturbances in pulmonary vasoregulation are more likely to be treated successfully by measures aimed directly at the pulmonary vasculature. Table 9.1 illustrates the spectrum of disturbances that occur in the pulmonary vasculature.

Management The management of elevated pulmonary vascular pressures and resistance postoperatively in the patient who has had cardiac surgery and is critically ill includes the following:

1. Sedation with major tranquilizers and narcotics
2. Optimizing oxygenation and ventilation (i.e., inducing a modest respiratory alkalosis)
3. Avoid excessive increases in airway pressures and air trapping

Table 9.1
Disturbances That Occur in the Pulmonary Vasculature

	PAP	PCWP	DP	CO	PVR
1	N	N	N	N	N
2	↑	↑	N	N/↓	N
3	↑	↑	↑	N/↓	N/↑
4	↑↑	↑	↑	↓	↑
5	↑	N/↑	↑↑	↓↓*	↑↑

*RV failure

PAP, Pulmonary Artery Pressure; *PCWP*, Pulmonary Capillary Wedge Pressure; *DP*, PAP−PCWP; *PVR*, Pulmonary Vascular Resistance; *N*, Normal

4. Inotropic support of right ventricular dysfunction; and if indicated
5. Pharmacological strategies that directly act on the pulmonary vessels, such as β-adrenergic agonists (e.g., isoproterenol), "intravenous nitric oxide donors" (i.e., nitroglycerin or sodium nitroprusside), milrinone, prostaglandin E-1 (infrequently used because of the concomitant need for systemic administration of α-adrenergic agonists to maintain systemic blood pressure), and inhaled nitric oxide. Potential future advances may include the use of inhaled prostacyclin in these patients.

Intra-Aortic Balloon Pump (IABP) An intra-aortic balloon pump (IABP) is a balloon on the end of a catheter which can be inflated/deflated cyclically using helium or CO_2. The catheter is 40 cm long, positioned in the aorta distal to the great vessels but proximal to the celiac plexus. An IABP is indicated if 1) left ventricular dysfunction is inadequately treated with drugs; or 2) ischemia is intractable to conventional medical treatment. The IABP increases the myocardial oxygen supply:demand ratio. Myocardial oxygen supply increases because the IABP inflates during ventricular diastole, the portion of the cardiac cycle when myocardial perfusion occurs. Inflation of the balloon displaces blood proximally toward the heart. As the aortic valve is closed during systole, the blood displaced toward the heart cannot enter the left ventricle and, instead, increases the pressure in the aortic root. By doing so, it increases the pressure in all arteries originating from the ascending and arch aorta, including the coronary arteries. This increase in coronary perfusion pressure effectively increases blood flow and oxygen supply to the myocardium. The IABP decreases myocardial oxygen demand by reducing left ventricular afterload. As the balloon inflates, blood is displaced distally in the descending thoracic aorta. This effectively decreases aortic pressure, promoting forward flow of blood in the aortic root when the balloon deflates immediately before ventricular systole.

An IABP is potentially useful any time the myocardial oxygen supply:demand ratio cannot be satisfactorily controlled by pharmacologic means (i.e., recalcitrant ischemia and cardiogenic shock). An IABP is most effective if these conditions are reversible (i.e., myocardial ischemia pre-CPB and viral myocarditis). It is not useful and is contraindicated in aortic valve incompetence and may be dangerous to use in severe atherosclerotic or aneurysmal disease of the aorta. Once an IABP is placed, there is the ongoing risk of occlusion of aortic great vessels (less likely if left radial pressure is not compromised) and gut ischemia, which is avoided by assuring proper position by locating the radio-opaque tip at the second or third intercostal space on CXR.

To be most effective, the timing of balloon inflation and deflation must be optimized. Appropriate inflation should begin at the moment of aortic valve closure, which is indicated in the aortic pressure tracing by the dicrotic notch and corresponds to a point midway through the T wave on EKG. Inflation beginning at this time results in a sharp "v"-shaped dicrotic notch followed by a pressure increase that peaks higher than the systolic pressure peak. Deflation should begin immediately before ventricular inflation, as indicated in the aortic pressure tracing at the point immediately preceding the beginning of the systolic pressure wave and corresponds to the R wave of the EKG.

Postoperative Bleeding and Cardiac Tamponade in the Cardiac Surgery Patient

The frequency of occurrence of significant postoperative bleeding and cardiac tamponade in patients after cardiac surgery is highly variable. Many factors influence the tendency to bleed:

1. Preoperative factors such as aspirin, oral anticoagulants, intravenous heparin, and thrombolytics
2. Liver disease
3. Renal disease
4. Platelet abnormalities

Intraoperative factors include the following:

1. Duration of cardiopulmonary bypass
2. Intraoperative use of aprotinin, platelets, and antifibrinolytics
3. Specific surgical procedure
4. Heparin rebound, acquired platelet defects, dilutional issues (platelets and factors), and fibrinolysis

The incidence of clinically significant bleeding postoperatively also depends on the endpoint used to define clinically significant bleeding (need for repeated blood transfusions versus need to return to the OR, etc.).

Cardiac tamponade occurs when blood accumulates in the pericardial sac, compressing the cardiac cavities and compromising cardiac output because of increasing filling pressures. The presence of fluid (usually blood) around the heart does not constitute cardiac tamponade. Tamponade has to include physiologic impairment of pump function as a result of pericardial fluid accumulation. It is not infrequent to have some pericardial fluid accumulation without hemodynamic compromise. This is best illustrated postoperatively in patients after cardiac transplant when a small heart is placed in a large pericardial sac, with nature abhorring the resultant cavity. The fluid accumulation in the pericardial sac may or may not result in tamponade.

Diagnosis of Cardiac Tamponade Cardiac tamponade is diagnosed by the presence of the following:

1. Increasing venous pressures
2. Decreasing cardiac output
3. Hypotension
4. Widening mediastinal shadow on chest x-ray
5. TEE (increase fluid in the pericardial sac with atrial compression)

Chest-tube output is not necessarily useful in establishing the presence or absence of cardiac tamponade. A decrease in chest-tube output could reflect continued bleeding with accumulation of pericardial blood, but also may reflect a decrease in bleeding. Likewise, continued chest-tube output might seem reassuring because it could indicate lack of pericardial fluid accumulation; however, this conclusion is contingent upon the belief that the whole pericardial sac is effectively drained. The accumulation of small amounts of blood (with or without clot) behind the atria (the low pressure chambers of the heart) may have significant hemodynamic consequences. Finally, a widening mediastinum demonstrated on chest x-ray and TEE (demonstrating pericardial fluid with or without atrial chamber compression) helps confirm the diagnosis of tamponade. Pericardial fluid on TEE without hemodynamic compromise or hemodynamic instability does not constitute a diagnosis of cardiac tamponade.

Management of Cardiac Tamponade

Management consists of the following:

1. Maintaining hemodynamics with volume (crystalloid, blood products, and blood), resuscitation, and inotropes
2. Diagnosis/treatment of medical bleeding (PT, PTT, platelet count, fibrinogen, fibrin split products, and directed replacement therapy)
3. Surgical exploration for relief of tamponade and for the identification/treatment of surgical sources of bleeding

Frequently, patients have both medical and surgical bleeding. Surgical reexploration of the mediastinal cavity in the operating room also is indicated (even in the absence of surgical bleeding) in patients whose medical bleeding causes hemodynamically significant compromise.

Pulmonary Ventilation/Oxygenation Issues Post-CPB

Ventilator Weaning

In patients after cardiac surgery who are routine and have no complications postoperatively, the inspired oxygen concentration is decreased as soon as possible (as indicated by the P_aO_2 or the O_2 saturation) after the patient has returned to the ICU. Mechanical respiratory support is weaned when the patient is warm and hemodynamically stable. Several factors specific to the patient who has had cardiac surgery contribute to protracted weaning and an increased A-a gradient including the following:

1. Effects of anesthesia with intubation decreasing FRC
2. Sternotomy
3. Surgical manipulation
4. Pleural fluid
5. Pain with splinting
6. Interstitial and alveolar fluid accumulation during and following CPB
7. Phrenic nerve damage with diaphragmatic dysfunction

These and other issues render the ventilatory management of even routine postoperative cardiac patients more problematic than that of noncardiac patients. Historically, such patients were extubated 12 to 24 hours postoperatively. However, contemporary factors have now conspired to attempt extubation in these patients as soon as they are normothermic, hemodynamically stable, demonstrate hemostasis, and are neurologically intact. This usually occurs 4 to 8 hours postoperatively.

Prolonged postoperative ventilatory support is common in this patient population because cardiac surgery with CPB results in specific changes that compromise both ventilation and oxygenation (vide supra). Moreover, the preoperative risk factors for cardiac disease (and thus cardiac surgery) are often identical to those for pulmonary disease (e.g., smoking). Factors associated with prolonged ventilation are outlined in Table 9.2. Management of these patients consist of 1) addressing the underlying causes (e.g., infection, cardiac failure, fluid overload, etc.); and 2) providing supportive respiratory care (bronchodilators, mucolytics, ventilator manipulation, etc.).

Postoperative Shivering

Cardiac patients have a progressive decrease in temperature for 1 to 2 hours postoperatively when cold, poorly perfused tissues reequilibrate with warm, well-perfused tissues. Shivering constitutes a normal body response to maintain normothermia and de-

Table 9.2
Factors Associated with Protracted Mechanical Ventilation After Cardiac Surgery

1. Respiratory	a. Preoperative compromised pulmonary function
	b. Bronchospasm
	c. Pulmonary hypertension
	d. Infection
	e. Phrenic nerve damage
2. Cardiovascular	a. Bleeding/tamponade/reoperation
	b. Poor left ventricular function
	c. Emergency procedure
	d. Fluid overload
3. Elderly patient	
4. Neurological injury	
5. Renal failure	

pends on an intact central thermoregulatory center and intact neuromuscular function. Shivering produces carbon dioxide and interferes with mechanical ventilation (if severe) and also requires increased myocardial and striated muscle oxygen absorption. Thus, patients are also at risk of myocardial ischemia. If shivering is not severe and the patient is hemodynamically stable, then the patient can be treated safely with meperidine (25 mg). If shivering is severe, it may require use of muscle relaxants (pancuronium and vecuronium). These should only be used if the patient is adequately sedated or anesthetized.

Renal/Fluid/Electrolyte Management

The Early Postoperative Period

Quantifying prior fluid deficit and ongoing losses immediately following cardiac surgery is difficult. It is nearly impossible to accurately determine blood loss and fluid administration during CPB. Furthermore, although fluid losses in the form of urine and drain output can be assessed easily, it is difficult to quantify third space losses. The capillary leak mediated by stress and CPB exposure varies in severity and duration, but tends to be proportional to the duration of CPB.

Urine output, though normally a good indication of volume status, can be deceptive in a patient after a bypass. Urine output can overestimate volume status because of residual effects of diuretics (mannitol/Lasix) given during CPB, and urine output can underestimate volume status in patients with good preoperative renal function who had ATN during CPB. This makes it important to use other parameters of adequate tissue perfusion (e.g., pedal pulses, capillary refill, and PA catheter) in assessing volume status immediately after CPB.

The fluid-seeking phase after CPB is short in duration, usually resolving in 6 to 12 hours. Much of the residual effects of diuretics typically given during CPB (mannitol/Lasix) also resolve over this period. Finally, hypothermia and the associated vasoconstriction usually have been corrected within 6 hours. Ongoing fluid requirements typically diminish after 6 to 12 hours in these patients. Therefore, fluid mobilization and diuresis become the focus of fluid and electrolyte management. The ability to manage fluid and electrolytes frequently is tempered by poor ventricular function and/or renal impairment. The inability to effect an adequate diuresis in these patients contributes to protracted respiratory support and care.

Oliguric renal failure is a serious complication postoperatively in cardiac patients, occurring in 2 to 4% of patients. Oliguric renal failure is associated with multiorgan failure and significant mortality. Factors associated with postoperative renal failure include the following:

1. Low cardiac output with the need for circulatory support
2. Preoperative cardiac failure
3. Preoperative elevated creatinine
4. Long CPB (± hemoglobinuria)
5. Blood transfusions
6. Postoperative hypotension and low cardiac output.

Optimizing urine output during CPB may be important in decreasing the incidence of renal failure. Mannitol administration during CPB is used almost universally, whereas the efficacy of dopamine is more controversial. Postoperative renal failure may demonstrate a spectrum of severity as listed:

1. Transient elevation of serum creatinine (no intervention required)
2. Renal failure requiring temporary CAVH/CVVH/dialysis
3. Protracted renal failure requiring long-term dialysis

Infections in Cardiac Surgery Patients

Pulmonary infections: septicemia, mediastinitis, or UTI are not uncommon after cardiac surgery. The predilection to these infections is related to the patient population and the surgery performed (sternotomy/mediastinitis, urinary catheter/UTI, etc.). The organisms involved reflect the environment, the antibiotics used perioperatively, and the source/port of entry for the infection. Treatment and overall management does not differ from that for patients who have had noncardiac surgery.

10

Pediatric Cardiac Intensive Care[1]

Keith C. Kocis

CARDIAC

Patient History

A complete history should be obtained on every child admitted to the cardiothoracic intensive care unit (CTICU). Specifically, the patient's diagnosis must be known in detail and the diagnostic evaluation (echocardiogram, cardiac catheterizations, electrophysiologic study, etc.) must be known in detail. The surgical history of a pediatric cardiac patient must be well known. Previous palliative or corrective operations, postoperative complications including airway difficulties or prolonged intubation, length of hospitalization, and previous sites of vascular access must be reviewed by the CTICU team. This information can alert the cardiac intensivists about potential problems that may complicate the present CTICU course. All present and previous medications and allergies should be identified. Other medical or surgical history should be elicited. Any recent illness (i.e., viral respiratory infection) also should be detailed in the history.

---

[1]Portions of this chapter were previously published and are reprinted with permission from Kocis K, Snikder AR. Congenital heart disease. In: Rakel RE, ed. Conn's current therapy. Philadelphia: W.B. Saunders, 1994;270–276.

Physical Examination

The weight of a child with congenital heart disease remains an important parameter to be measured and monitored. Ideally, the child's weight, height, and head circumference should be plotted against age, and data since birth should be available. This will provide an overall assessment of the child's growth and nutritional status prior to operation. In children that are not thriving, the weight is disproportionately less than height. Head circumference is the last growth parameter to fall off the growth curve. Acute weight gain is often associated with acute congestive heart failure. In the immediate perioperative period, the weight of the child aids in fluid management. To obtain reliable and reproducible data, the weight should be obtained using a strict and consistent protocol. Postoperatively, the growth parameters should normalize in children who have undergone complete repair of their lesions. In children who continue to lag, significant residual lesions or other etiologies should be sought.

During the physical examination, particular attention must be given to the child's vital signs (including four-limb blood pressure measurements), general appearance (cyanotic versus acyanotic, well nourished versus wasted), state (comfortable, distressed, shock), cardiac findings, pulmonary signs (depth and rate of breathing, use of accessory respiratory muscles, presence of rales), abdominal examination (location and size of liver and location of stomach), femoral pulses (intensity and presence of radial-femoral delay), and distal extremities (temperature, cyanosis, clubbing, edema).

The cardiac examination should proceed serially and methodically with inspection, palpation, percussion, and auscultation, but is often limited in the postoperative period because of the presence of bandages, tubes, and noises in the CTICU. When auscultating the pediatric heart, the quality of the first and second heart sounds and the presence of the third or fourth heart sounds should be noted. The second heart sound should be analyzed closely noting its variation with respiration. Systolic murmurs are quantified on a scale of 1 to 6 with murmurs of grade 4 or above associated with the presence of a thrill. Regurgitant (holosystolic) murmurs begin with the first heart sound and, therefore, obscure it, whereas ejection murmurs begin after the first heart sound. Diastolic murmurs are quantified on a scale of 1 to 4 with grade 4 murmurs associated with the presence of a thrill. Continuous murmurs extend through both systole and diastole. Localization of the murmurs to the classic mitral, tricuspid, aortic, and pulmonic areas is helpful. Additionally, auscultation over the posterior thorax bilaterally and supraclavicular regions is necessary.

Cyanosis is detected clinically when 3 g/dL of desaturated hemoglobin is present. Central cyanosis, best seen in the tongue and buccal mucosa, must be differentiated from acrocyanosis (peripheral). Noninvasive pulse oximetry is most useful for diagnosing and quantifying cyanosis. Typically, the oxygen saturation should be greater than 90% in neonates and 95% in infants and children.

Major Cardiac Lesions

Most forms of CHD can be categorized into 1) *Acyanotic CHD* subdivided into groups with increased pulmonary vascularity or ventricular outflow obstruction or; 2) *Cyanotic CHD* subdivided into groups with decreased pulmonary vascularity or increased pulmonary vascularity. Patients can be appropriately categorized into the above groups and a presumptive diagnosis is made by integrating information obtained from the physical examination, chest radiograph, and pulse oximeter.

Acyanotic CHD with Increased Pulmonary Vascularity

Several congenital heart defects present with acyanosis and increased pulmonary vascularity. The most common defects in this category are as follows:

1. Ventricular septal defect
2. Atrial septal defect
3. Patent ductus arteriosus
4. Atrioventricular septal defect

In total, these four lesions account for the majority of CHD (50%).

Ventricular Septal Defect (VSD). VSD is the most common form of CHD occurring in 32% of children with heart disease. The ventricular septum is a complex structure described embryologically as having four major regions:

1. Inlet septum located posteriorly and superiorly between the tricuspid and mitral valves
2. Outlet septum located anteriorly beneath the aortic and pulmonary valves
3. Trabecular septum located inferiorly
4. Membranous septum located in the subaortic region and beneath the septal leaflet of the tricuspid valve

The largest part of the ventricular septum is the trabecular region, and fusion of the inlet, outlet, and trabecular septa occurs in the membranous region.

Patients with a VSD have a dependent left-to-right shunt, meaning that the relative pressures and resistances of both the systemic and pulmonary circulations determine the amount and direction of ventricular level shunting. At birth, when the pulmonary vascular pressures and resistances are high, little left-to-right ventricular shunting occurs. During the first 2 to 6 weeks of life, pulmonary pressures and vascular resistances decrease, creating a pressure difference between the left and right ventricles and, therefore, allowing shunting from left to right. The amount of ventricular shunting is also dependent on the size of the VSD, with larger defects allowing more blood to shunt. In addition, other associated cardiac lesions may alter the amount and direction of shunting.

The clinical signs and symptoms of children with VSD are the result of the amount of left-to-right ventricular shunting. Neonates are often without symptomatology, and only as pulmonary pressures and vascular resistances decrease do clinical symptoms develop.

Eisenmenger syndrome develops when a large VSD is unrepaired and pulmonary hypertension and irreversible pulmonary vascular obstructive disease develops, resulting in right-to-left ventricular shunting and cyanosis. Death follows as a result of pulmonary hemorrhage, infections, and/or paradoxical emboli.

With advances in the medical and surgical care of children with CHD, cardiothoracic surgery is now being performed safely, even in small infants. Indications for surgical closure of a VSD include the following:

1. Uncontrolled congestive heart failure
2. Increased pulmonary vascular resistance with a risk for development of pulmonary vascular obstructive disease
3. Inability to thrive despite maximum medical therapy
4. Recurrent pulmonary infections
5. Endocarditis
6. Paradoxical emboli

Atrial Septal Defect (ASD). ASD is the third most common form of CHD occurring in 8% of children with heart disease. ASD is found more frequently in females than males (2:1).

ASDs occur in three locations in the atrial septum. Ostium primum defects are located in the lower third of the atrial septum near the atrioventricular valves. Ostium secundum defects are found in the mid portion of the septum. Sinus venosus defects occur in the posterior portion of the septum adjacent to the vena cavae. Ostium secundum defects are the most common.

The direction and amount of atrial level shunting is determined by the relative compliances of the right and left ventricles and the size of the defect. Typically, the right ventricle is more compliant and, therefore, predominantly left-to-right shunting occurs.

Indications for closure of an ASD are as follows:

1. Right ventricular volume overload
2. Arrhythmias
3. Paradoxical emboli
4. Elevated pulmonary vascular resistance

Closure is performed surgically with little morbidity or mortality.

Patent Ductus Arteriosus (PDA). Approximately 2% of children with CHD have an isolated PDA. Premature infants have a high incidence of PDA, which is inversely proportional to their gestational age. The ductus arteriosus is a normal embryological structure connecting the main pulmonary artery to the descending aorta. In normal term infants, this structure closes within the first few days of life. Patients with a PDA have left-to-right shunting dependent on the size of the PDA and pressures in the descending aorta and pulmonary artery.

Indomethacin successfully closes most PDAs in premature infants and surgical closure is only occasionally necessary. Surgical ligation is extremely effective with essentially no morbidity or mortality in older children.

Atrioventricular Septal Defect (AVSD). AVSD occurs in 7% of children with CHD and is common in children with Down syndrome. The defect is comprised of a large defect in the atrioventricular septum along with a common atrioventricular valve. To avoid acute and long-term consequences of pulmonary hypertension, surgical repair is required in infancy, ideally at 3 to 6 months of age.

Acyanotic CHD with Ventricular Outflow Tract Obstruction

Ventricular outflow tract obstruction can occur in both the left and right ventricles. Obstruction to either ventricle can be isolated or in combination with other defects at the subvalvar, valvar, or supravalvar levels.

Aortic Stenosis (AS). AS occurs in 3% of children with CHD. The commissures of the aortic valve are fused, resulting in a thickened, domed, and stenotic orifice. The symptoms and findings on physical examination are variable and relate to the degree of narrowing of the valve.

Surgery is recommended for those in whom the annulus and valve are very small, requiring valve replacement or in whom balloon valvuloplasty was unsuccessful.

Coarctation of the Aorta (CoA). CoA occurs in 5% of children with CHD. CoA is a constriction of the descending aorta that usually occurs opposite the ductus/ligamentum arteriosus. The symptomatology in these patients is variable. Typically, children with mild disease have no symptoms, whereas infants with critical CoA present with shock in the first week of life after spontaneous closure of the ductus arteriosus. Prostaglandin E_1 infusion is lifesaving for neonates with critical CoA in shock because of its ability to open and maintain the patency of the ductus arteriosus and, therefore, allow blood flow into the descending aorta. Most children with CoA undergo surgical repair. Many children with CoA have postoperative hypertension that usually is controlled well with beta receptor blockade.

Pulmonic Stenosis (PS). PS is the second most common form of CHD occurring in 9% of children with heart disease. The pulmonary valve is abnormal with fusion of the commissures, resulting in a thickened, domed, and stenotic orifice. Balloon valvuloplasty is usually successful in treating this lesion. Surgery is contemplated only in children with severely dysplastic and hypoplastic valves or those with additional obstruction at the subvalvar or supravalvar locations.

Cyanotic CHD with Decreased Pulmonary Vascularity

Patients with cyanotic CHD and decreased pulmonary vascularity have obstructed pulmonary blood flow and right-to-left shunting of blood either at the atrial or ventricular level. In the neonatal period, children with this category of defects are usually intensely cyanotic with hyperpnea but not dyspnea. This presentation is because of the decrease in pulmonary blood flow and absence of congestive heart failure.

Tetralogy of Fallot (TOF). TOF is the most common form of cyanotic CHD occurring in 7% of children with CHD. The tetralogy consists of the following:

1. Pulmonary stenosis (subvalvar, valvar, supravalvar)
2. VSD
3. Aorta overriding the ventricular septum
4. Right ventricular hypertrophy

Patients present with a varying degree of cyanosis dependent on the severity of the pulmonary stenosis. A hypercyanotic spell or "tetralogy spell" is a characteristic sequence of clinical events that begins with irritability and hyperpnea followed by a prolonged period of intense cyanosis leading to syncope.

Medical treatment is lifesaving in children with a hypercyanotic spell. Initially, the child should be calmed and comforted and placed in a knee-to-the-chest position. Maximal supplemental oxygen by face mask is then given. If the spell continues, morphine is given intramuscularly at a dose of 0.1 mg/kg. If the spell persists, then more aggressive therapy is initiated. This includes rapid placement of an intravenous catheter by the most experienced personnel followed by intravenous fluid administration (10 to 20 mL/kg of 0.9% saline) and sodium bicarbonate administration (1 mEq/kg). Anemia (hemoglobin less than 10 g/dL) when present, often precipitates a hypercyanotic spell, and blood transfusion may be required.

Surgical repair of this defect is indicated for any child with hypercyanotic spells or increasing cyanosis (typically oxygen saturation less than 75%). Until recently, the approach to these patients had been a palliative operation involving placement of a modified Blalock-Taussig shunt (Gore-tex tube connection between the innominate artery and pulmonary artery) in infancy followed by definitive repair (pulmonary valvotomy with resection of right ventricular infundibular muscle bundles and VSD closure) in older childhood (age 3 to 4 years). With advancements in the combined medical and surgical management of younger infants, definitive repair often is being performed in infancy as the only surgical procedure.

Tricuspid Atresia (TA). TA is a rare form of CHD in which the tricuspid valve orifice is not patent. A patent foramen ovale or ASD is present to allow systemic venous blood to shunt from right to left. The right ventricle and pulmonary outflow tract are typically hypoplastic, unless a large VSD is present. These patients present in the immediate neonatal period with significant cyanosis. Initial medical therapy includes the initiation of prostaglandin E_1 infusion (0.05 μg/kg per minute) to maintain the patency of the ductus arteriosus. Palliative surgery is performed in the first week of life and consists of placement of a modified Blalock-Taussig shunt. A modified bidirectional Glenn anastomosis connecting the superior vena cava to the top of the right pulmonary artery is performed at 6 to 9 months as a staged approach followed by the modified Fontan operation at approximately 2 years of age. The modified Fontan operation allows complete bypass of the right side of the heart by directing inferior and superior vena cavae flow into the pulmonary arteries.

Cyanotic CHD with Increased Pulmonary Vascularity

Cardiac lesions with cyanosis and increased pulmonary vascularity can be divided further into those with increased pulmonary 1) arterial (transposition of the great arteries and truncus arteriosus); or 2) venous vascularity (total anomalous pulmonary venous connection and hypoplastic left heart syndrome).

Transposition of the Great Arteries (TGA). In TGA, the aorta rises from the right ventricle while the pulmonary artery rises from the left ventricle. The pulmonary and systemic circulations are configured in parallel rather than in series, resulting in cyanotic blood recirculating back to the systemic circulation. Medical management involves stabilizing the neonate and initiating a prostaglandin E_1 infusion (0.05 μg/kg per minute) while awaiting balloon septostomy. The infants are stabilized after balloon septostomy and undergo surgical repair of the defect in the first week of life. The arterial switch operation, in which the aorta is connected to the left ventricle and the pulmonary artery to the right ventricle with transfer of the coronary arteries, is now the surgical procedure of choice.

Truncus arteriosus (TR). TR is a rare form of CHD whereby a single valved vessel is located above both right and left ventricles with a large VSD allowing for common egress of blood from both ventricles. This common vessel, the truncus arteriosus, gives rise to the aorta, coronary arteries, and pulmonary arteries. A significant percentage of these patients have DiGeorge Sequence (thymic hypoplasia, third and fourth pharyngeal pouch syndrome) and should be evaluated immediately for hypocalcemia secondary to hypoparathyroidism and T-cell immunodeficiency. These patients should receive only irradiated blood cell transfusions to prevent graft versus host disease. Definitive surgical repair usually can be performed soon after diagnosis and involves placement of a valved homograft conduit from the right ventricle to the main pulmonary artery that has been separated from the truncus arteriosus. The VSD is closed to direct the left ventricular blood into the truncus arteriosus. Subsequent surgical procedures are necessary to change the size of the conduit as the children grow.

Total Anomalous Pulmonary Venous Connection (TAPVC). Patients with TAPVC, a rare form of CHD, have their entire supply of oxygenated pulmonary venous blood returning to the systemic venous circulation. This mixture of oxygenated and desaturated blood produces cyanosis. The severity of the cyanosis increases if there is an obstruction to the return of the pulmonary venous blood, which is common. Neonates with TAPVC frequently present in extremis with severe cyanosis. Surgical repair is done immediately on presentation with good long-term results.

Hypoplastic Left Heart Syndrome (HLHS). HLHS occurs in 4% of children with CHD and is comprised of stenosis or atresia of the mitral and/or aortic valves, CoA, and hypoplasia of the left ventricle. Neonates present within the first few days of life, typically with mild cyanosis and shock after the PDA begins to close. Initial medical management is lifesaving. Control of the airway and mechanical ventilation are necessary. Prostaglandin E_1 infusion (0.05 μg/kg per minute) is initiated and the state of shock is treated with fluid administration (bolus 10 to 20 mL/kg of 0.9% saline or 5% albumin) and inotropic support (dopamine infusion of 3 to 10 μg/kg per minute). Surgical treatment for this disease is variable and controversial. In some centers, no therapy is offered and the neonates die after intensive support is withdrawn. Cardiac transplantation at a few centers has had success, but the limited number of donor organs and life-long immunosuppression are of major concern. Select quaternary care centers use a staged surgical approach similar to that for children with TA. With this approach, neonates undergo the palliative Norwood operation (anastomosis of the divided main pulmonary artery to the aorta, aortic arch reconstruction, atrial septectomy, modified Blalock-Taussig shunt). This procedure transforms the right ventricle into the single pumping chamber for both the systemic circulation and, via the shunt, the pulmonary circulation. At 3 to 6 months, the infant proceeds to the bidirectional Glenn operation with removal of the Blalock-Taussig shunt followed by the modified Fontan operation at 2 years.

PULMONARY

Airway

Airway management of the child with congenital heart disease in the perioperative period is critically important and is the primary focus for the cardiac intensivist. Intubation should be performed only by personnel skilled in pediatric airway management. There are some general principles to follow; however, specific situations require deviation from this plan. Preparation is the key element for successful intubation. A variety of laryngoscope blades should be available for intubating infants and children of all ages. Commonly used blades are a 0-Miller for neonates, 1-Miller for young infants (1 to 6 months), 2-Macintosh/Miller for children (6 months to 6 years) and 3-Macintosh for older children (more than 6 years) and adolescents. A full array of endotracheal tubes including cuffed tubes are needed. The size of the endotracheal tube is approximated by the formula: (16 + age in years) / 4. Most term neonates can be intubated with a 3.5 mm tube. A stylet is helpful for smaller infants. An appropriate fitting mask with bag and suction is required. Preoxygenation with 100% oxygen is necessary for most infants except those with pulmonary overcirculation (i.e., hypoplastic left heart syndrome) in whom less oxygen is necessary to prevent a further decrease in systemic circulation. The intubation drugs used must have stable hemodynamic properties. Atropine is used for most children except those in which tachycardia would produce an unacceptable increase in myocardial oxygen demand (i.e., anomalous left coronary artery); glycopyrrolate should be used for these patients. Narcotics are the mainstay of analgesia for cardiac patients. Fentanyl is more potent than morphine and does not release histamine, which can result in hypotension. Short-acting benzodiazepines are excellent anxiolytics and work synergistically with narcotics. Ketamine can be used in patients who can not tolerate any degree of hypotension (i.e., coronary artery fistula). Ketamine results in an increase in systemic vascular resistance, blood pressure, and cardiac output by releasing epinephrine despite a direct negative effect on contractility. The increase in cardiac output is seen in all patients except those who are chronically stressed and, therefore, depleted in epinephrine stores. Ketamine should not be used in patients with pulmonary hypertension because it also increases pulmonary vascular resistance. Barbiturates cause unacceptable hypotension, decreased cardiac contractility, and should not be used in cardiac patients. Etomidate is a new anesthetic agent that produces rapid unconsciousness and is extremely cardiac stable. Experience with this drug is developing in children. Paralytic agents can be used for complete control of the airway. Succinylcholine, a short-acting depolarizing neuromuscular blocker, can be used only with caution because it causes potassium release that may provoke arrhythmias. Rocuronium, a new nondepolarizing neuromuscular blocker with rapid onset of action may be useful for cardiac patients. Vecuronium is a nondepolarizing neuromuscular blocker that has the most stable cardiac effects and commonly is used in cardiac patients. It does not have a rapid onset of action, limiting its use for rapid sequence intubations.

Oxygen Therapy

The inspired fraction of oxygen (F_IO_2) should be adjusted depending on the specific lesion, recognizing that oxygen (O_2) is a potent pulmonary vasodilator and causes acute lung injury at high concentrations. In children with pulmonary overcirculation (i.e., VSD), the F_IO_2 should be as low as possible to prevent a further decrease in pulmonary vascular resistance resulting in increased pulmonary overcirculation, while maintaining adequate O_2 saturation at 90 to 94%. In children with cyanotic lesions, the F_IO_2 should be titrated to the lowest value that produces the highest oxygen saturation, recognizing that many cyanotic lesions with fixed pulmonary blood flow will not respond to increased F_IO_2. In children with unrepaired hypoplastic left heart syndrome, F_IO_2 more than 21% can increase pulmonary circulation and decrease systemic blood flow, which can be lethal. Finally, in acute congestive heart failure (i.e., cardiomyopathy), the F_IO_2 should be as high as necessary to maintain O_2 saturation more than 95% to maximize oxygen delivery.

Ventilatory Support

Mechanical ventilatory support for a child after cardiac surgery must be tailored to the specific lesion and respiratory management goals. New ventilators are available that allow for easy patient triggering (either pressure or flow triggering) with rapid response times and small measurable and deliverable tidal volumes. This permits most neonates to trigger and ventilate in a volume-limited mode. Volume limiting is preferable in cardiac patients because the minute ventilation (tidal volume × respiratory rate) that is delivered is fixed. This is critically important because lung-compliance is often changing rapidly, which in a pressure limited mode results in a fluctuating tidal volume, minute ventilation, and therefore, $PaCO_2$ and pH. This can result in respiratory acidosis (decreased compliance with a decreased tidal volume and minute ventilation) or volutrauma (increased compliance with an increased tidal volume and minute ventilation). The alteration in $PaCO_2$ and pH, results in changes in pulmonary vascular resistance that can be extremely detrimental. Asynchronous, pressure-limited, continuous-flow ventilators without pressure-support options are no longer acceptable in a pediatric cardiac intensive care unit. Pressure-limited ventilation is used when lung compliance is so poor that the peak inspiratory pressure exceeds 30 to 35 mm Hg. This limits further barotrauma to the patient's lungs.

The three phases of respiratory support for children after cardiac surgery include the following:

1. Preoperative stabilization
2. Immediate postoperative stabilization
3. Weaning from mechanical ventilation

In the preoperative period, the goal of ventilatory support is to optimize the patient's ventilation and oxygenation and decrease the work of breathing. This can be obtained by ventilating the child in a synchronized intermittent mandatory ventilatory mode (SIMV) that is volume-limited (15 to 20 mL/kg total or 8 to 10 mL/kg corrected for compressible volume) at modest rates (infants = 20 to 25; children = 15 to 20; adolescents = 10 to 12). Pressure support is set to deliver 6 to 8 mL/kg total tidal volume and should be added to assist any spontaneous respirations above the mandatory rate. Positive end-expiratory pressure (PEEP) is set at 3 to 5 cm H_20 except in children and adolescents with decreased lung compliance who may require more.

In the immediate postoperative period, the goal of ventilatory support is to optimize the patient's ventilation and oxygenation, decrease the work of breathing, and maximize the patient's cardiac output with appropriate ventilatory settings. This can be obtained by ventilating the child in a controlled ventilatory mode that is volume-limited (15 to 20 mL/kg or 8 to 10 mL/kg corrected for compressible volume) at modest rates (infants = 20 to 25; children = 15 to 20; adolescents = 10 to 12). PEEP is set at 3 to 5 cm H_2O. Higher levels of PEEP decrease left ventricular afterload, but also decrease venous return to the heart (preload). Lower levels of PEEP (2 cm H_2O) are necessary for patients who have passive pulmonary blood flow (i.e., after a Bidirectional Glenn or Fontan operation). The inspiratory time should not be prolonged because this also can decrease venous return to the heart (preload). Typical inspiratory times are as follows: infants = 0.5 to 0.6 seconds; children = 0.7 to 1 second; adolescents = 1 second.

When weaning from mechanical ventilation, the goal of ventilatory support is to optimize the patient's ventilation and oxygenation and increase the work of breathing. This can be obtained by ventilating the child in a SIMV mode that is volume-limited (15 to 20 mL/kg total or 8 to 10 mL/kg corrected for compressible volume) at progressively lower backup rates. Pressure support is set to deliver 6 to 8 mL/kg total tidal volume and is added to assist all spontaneous breaths above the mandatory rate. Patients also can be weaned in a straight pressure support or volume support mode. Patients should have stable hemodynamics, stable airway, appropriate leak around the endotracheal tube (< 30 cm H_2O), normal static lung compliance (2 to 4 mL/cm H_2O), minimal excess chest wall edema, scant secretions, no atelectasis, no respiratory distress, no gastric dilation, controlled pain, and an alert state. Extubation can proceed with appropriate equipment and personnel available in the event of failed extubation trial. PEEP is set at 3 to 5 cm H_2O except in patients with passive pulmonary blood flow.

Pharmacologic Support for Cardiac Failure

There are both parasympathetic and sympathetic nervous system inputs to the heart and vasculature regulating heart rate, contractility, stroke volume, cardiac output, blood pressure, and systemic and pulmonary resistances. The vagus nerve (CN X) innervates the heart by using acetylcholine as the active neurotransmitter (both pre- and postganglionic neurons). The sympathetic nervous system innervates the heart by the cervical ganglia, and ganglia from thoracic levels 1 to 4. The preganglionic neurotransmitter is acetylcholine whereas the post ganglionic transmitter is norepinephrine. In addition, sympathetic inputs to the adrenal glands travel via the greater splanchnic nerve.

Adrenoreceptors

Classically described, there are α, β, and Dopaminergic receptors present throughout the body. α-Receptors are subdivided into α1-

and α2-receptors and are activated by norepinephrine and epinephrine. α1-Receptors located at the neuromuscular junction cause vasoconstriction on the vasculature whereas those located on the myocardium increase contractility. α2-Receptors located on presynaptic neurons are inhibitory, resulting in a decrease in norepinephrine release and therefore vasodilatation. This provides a negative feedback loop. α2-Receptors are found peripherally on smooth muscle causing vasoconstriction when stimulated. Because these receptors are found distant from the neuromuscular junction, they are thought to be stimulated by circulating epinephrine only. Lastly, there are central α2-receptors located within the medulla of the brainstem. When stimulated, these receptors are inhibitory, decreasing sympathetic output.

β-Receptors are divided into β1-receptors (cardiac) and β2-receptors (vascular/bronchial). β1-Receptors are stimulated by epinephrine, norepinephrine, dopamine, dobutamine, and isoproterenol. Stimulation of these receptors results in an increase in heart rate, contractility, stroke volume, and cardiac index. β2-Receptors are stimulated by epinephrine and isoproterenol, but not norepinephrine. When stimulated, the β2-receptor decreases blood pressure and systemic vascular resistance and causes bronchodilation.

Dopamine (DA 1) receptors are found on the renal, coronary, splanchnic, cerebral, and pulmonary (few) beds. Stimulation of this receptor results in vasodilation. DA 2 receptors are found on preganglionic neurons, are inhibitory in function, and decrease the release of norepinephrine, providing a negative feedback loop. Lastly, central dopamine receptors are found within the brain inhibiting the release of prolactin, thyrotropin, growth hormone, and gonadotropins.

Catecholamines are synthesized from the amino acid, tyrosine, serially into DOPA, dopamine, and norepinephrine. In the adrenal gland, norepinephrine is converted into epinephrine. Catecholamines are degraded by two major pathways: COMT (catechol-O-methyl transferase) and MAO (monamine oxidase). In addition, complex regulation of catecholamines occurs via reuptake of norepinephrine within the synapse and down regulation and sequestration of receptors.

Dopamine is an endogenous catecholamine with $t_{1/2}$ β of 6.9

minutes in neonates and 26 minutes in children. Its action may be prolonged with renal and or liver failure. Dose-related effects are found in children. At a dose of 0.5 to 2 μg/kg per minute, the effects are dopaminergic. At a higher dose of 2 to 5 μg/kg per minute the effects are β1. Finally, at doses of 5 to 20 μg/kg per minute, α1 effects are seen. The major side effects with dopamine use are tachyarrhythmias and tissue necrosis when extravasated. 75% of intravenous dopamine is metabolized by kidney, liver, and plasma (mostly MAO), whereas 25% is converted to norepinephrine in neurons for subsequent release. 50% of the cardiovascular effects of dopamine are by an indirect release of norepinephrine at the neuromuscular junction. If patients are chronically stressed and depleted of norepinephrine, dopamine is a much less effective inotrope.

Dobutamine is a synthetic catecholamine with a $t_{1/2}$ β of 26 minutes in children. Its half-life is significantly decreased when dopamine is simultaneously infused. Dobutamine is metabolized by COMT and no significant delays in metabolism are found with renal or hepatic failure. Usual dose range is 2 to 20 μg/kg per minute for β1 effects.

Isoproterenol is a synthetic catecholamine with β1 and β2 effects resulting in an increase in heart rate, contractility, stroke volume, and cardiac index and a decrease in systemic vascular resistance, pulmonary vascular resistance, and blood pressure. Isoproterenol is a potent bronchodilator. The $t_{1/2}$ β is 3 minutes in children. Isoproterenol is metabolized by COMT. The major side effects found are tachyarrhythmias, decreased myocardial oxygen consumption, and hypoxia secondary to ventilation-perfusion mismatch.

Epinephrine is an endogenous catecholamine with a $t_{1/2}$ β of 2 minutes. Its effects in children are dose-related with β1, 2 effects seen at doses of 0.01 to 0.08 μg/kg per minute, resulting in a decrease in SVR and PVR. At doses of 0.08 to 3 μg/kg per minute, α1, 2 effects are seen. The major side effects are tachyarrhythmias.

Norepinephrine is an endogenous catecholamine with a $t_{1/2}$ β of 2 minutes. Norepinephrine results in the stimulation of α1, 2 and β1-adrenoreceptors. This results in an increase in HR, contractility, stroke volume, CI, BP, SVR, PVR. The typical dose range is 0.05 to 2 μg/kg per minute with major side effects being tachyarrhythmias and decreased renal perfusion.

Amrinone and milrinone are both bipyridines, which is a new noncatecholamine class of inotrope. Bypyridines are selective inhibitors of cyclic nucleotide phosphodiesterase III leading to increases in cAMP and intracellular calcium. This results in an increase in contractility, stroke volume, and CI, and decreasing SVR and PVR. Amrinone has a $t_{1/2}$ β of 14 hours in neonates, 4 hours in older infants and children, and 8 hours in adults. It is principally metabolized by liver acetylation and is excreted in the urine. An initial loading dose of 0.75 to 3 mg/kg is given followed by infusion at a rate of 2 to 20 μg/kg per minute. Typical side effects encountered are hypotension, requiring volume administration and thrombocytopenia.

Milrinone is similar to amrinone but is more potent. The $t_{1/2}$ β of milrinone is 2 hours. An initial loading dose of 50 μg/kg is given slowly followed by an infusion of 0.1 to 0.75 μg/kg per minute. Hypotension is a common side effect.

Calcium is the final metabolite for cardiac contraction. In the body, calcium is both free (ionized) and bound. Infusion of albumin, plasma, or citrate (an anticoagulant in packed red blood cells), decreases ionized calcium. Ionized calcium levels should be monitored closely (4.4 to 5.4 mg/dL; 1 to 1.35 mmol/L) and replaced with the chloride salt at a dose of 10 to 20 mg/kg intravenously. A continuous infusion can be administered at a dose of 1 to 5 mg/kg per hour in unstable postoperative patients. The major side effects are tissue necrosis when extravasated, so $CaCl_2$ should be administered through a patent central venous line.

Cardiac Evaluation

Electrocardiogram

An electrocardiogram should be obtained preoperatively and in select patients postoperatively. Any patient with suspicion of an arrhythmia warrants full investigation. Rate, rhythm, axis, intervals, hypertrophy, and ischemic changes should be evaluated. In addition, the ability to obtain atrial electrograms from either surgically placed atrial wires or from a transesophageal lead is a must.

Echocardiography

Echocardiography has become the principle method for diagnosing almost every form of congenital heart disease. Cardiac catheterization is no longer necessary for diagnosing most lesions. In addition, physiologic data can be obtained easily. Many indices, such as cardiac output, ventricular systolic and diastolic function, pressure gradients across stenotic valves, and pulmonary artery systolic and diastolic pressure, can be obtained. A load-independent measure of left ventricular systolic function (wall stress − velocity of circumferential fiber-shortening relationship) can be obtained using advanced echocardiographic principles. Imaging in the cardiac ICU can be difficult because of the multiple tubes, lines, incisions, bandages, etc.; therefore, transesophageal echocardiography must be readily available.

M-Mode. M-mode (motion-mode) echocardiography is an older technique that is still used today for precisely measuring endocardial borders when measuring the ventricular shortening fraction. It also is used to measure the velocity of circumferential fiber shortening. These measures are important to the intensivist interested in evaluating ventricular function.

Two-Dimensional Imaging. High-resolution imaging with small, lightweight, high-frequency transducers and advanced technology has enabled pediatric cardiologists to accurately visualize and diagnose complex congenital cardiac defects. The intensivist uses this modality to identify residual anatomic defects, pericardial or pleural effusions, cardiac vegetations, location of monitoring lines, paralyzed hemidiaphragms, and to calculate an ejection fraction (one estimate of ventricular systolic function).

Doppler Ultrasound Evaluation. Doppler echocardiography is a noninvasive method for measuring the velocity of red blood cells. The technique is extremely useful for calculating pressure gradients across stenotic valves using the modified Bernoulli equation (Δ Pressure $= 4 \times$ peak Velocity^2), estimating cardiac output (mean velocity $\times$ cross-sectional area of the valve), estimating pulmonary artery systolic pressure (via tricuspid regurgitation jets), pulmonary artery diastolic pressure (via pulmonary artery regurgitation jets), and assessing left ventricular diastolic function.

Color Doppler Ultrasound Evaluation. Color Doppler techniques supplement the previously mentioned diagnostic techniques, often increasing the sensitivity and accuracy of the complete ultrasound examination.

Dobutamine Stress Echocardiography. Dobutamine stress testing has become increasingly useful in diagnosing regional wall abnormalities within the left ventricle. Pediatric use is limited but increasing.

Peripheral Vascular Imaging. Imaging the major arteries and veins cannulated by intensivists can be done with the appropriate vascular probes. This is helpful in assessing a priori the patency of major vessels. When vascular thrombosis occurs, often a rapid diagnosis can be made.

Cardiac Catheterizations

Previous Catheterizations. With the increased number and complexity of interventional cardiac catheterizations in children, all intensivists must have a basic understanding of what can be accomplished in the catheterization laboratory. Cannulated vessels and unsuccessful cannulation sites should be known so that vessel cannulation in the ICU can be more successful. In addition, arterial obstructions (i.e., femoral artery) should be identified so that monitoring is performed in other sites.

Cardiac Catheterization. Cardiac catheterization has been transformed in the past decade. This procedure is performed increasingly for interventional procedures and less frequently for anatomic diagnosis. Hemodynamic assessment remains an important part of the pediatric cardiac catheterization. Oxygen saturation and pressures are recorded in all chambers of the heart, and oxygen consumption is measured directly. The calculations that are made include systemic and pulmonary blood flow, intracardiac shunts, systemic and pulmonary resistance, and oxygen delivery and extraction. Interventional procedures have evolved for balloon dilatation of semilunar valves, coarctation of the aorta, and branch pulmonary artery stenosis. Coil embolization of aortopulmonary collaterals and patent ductus arteriosus are now common. Device closure of atrial and ventricular defects are still experimental. Electrophysiologic investigation with mapping and ablation is common for diagnosing and treating arrhythmias in children.

Radiographic Evaluation

The chest radiograph is essential in the care of the pediatric cardiac ICU patient. Radiographs should be obtained daily in the immediate postoperative period. When patients are decompensating, a chest radiograph also should be obtained. The following information should be confirmed systematically: endotracheal tube position, proper central venous line positioning, placement of nasogastric tube, positioning of mediastinal and chest tubes, cardiac silhouette and size, side of aortic arch, lung aeration and evaluation of atelectasis, infiltrates, pulmonary edema, pneumothoraces, and pleural effusions. The chest radiograph must be compared with the preoperative study and to previous daily radiographs. Decubitus films help assess the size of pleural effusions. Injection of central venous lines with nonionic contrast can be performed at the bedside to assure intravascular placement.

Barium upper-gastrointestinal series are rarely performed for patients in the cardiac ICU. They are useful in assessing vascular rings preoperatively and in evaluating malrotation in patients with heterotaxy.

Fluoroscopy can be useful in assessing diaphragm motion and diagnosing a paralyzed hemidiaphragm. Portable fluoroscopy can be helpful for the placement of Swan-Ganz catheters in difficult patients.

Computer-aided tomography (CAT) of the chest is used infrequently but can be useful in diagnosing mediastinal abscesses and airway compression. Patients with an abnormal neurologic examination in whom a cerebral vascular accident is suspected are imaged rapidly with a CAT scan.

Magnetic resonance imaging (MRI) is used for the preoperative diagnose of complex congenital heart disease. In particular, pulmonary artery abnormalities and aortic arch anomalies are visualized easily using MRI. Rarely is the MRI used in the immediate postoperative period.

Thallium scanning is used to diagnose areas of nonviable, unperfused myocardium. This study is useful in diagnosing myocardial injury in patients with coronary anomalies (anomalous left coronary artery, Kawasaki's disease, etc.).

MUGA scans are used to assess left ventricular systolic function. First Pass angiocardiography is used to assess extra- and intracardiac shunting.

Ventilation Perfusion Scan (V/Q) scans can be helpful in diagnosing pulmonary embolism and ventilation–perfusion mismatch.

Arrhythmias

Arrhythmia management has become increasingly common in the pediatric cardiothoracic ICU because of the treatment and survival of children with complex congenital heart disease. Normal reference values for heart rate and the ECG intervals should be readily accessible in the CTICU because they are age-dependent

Bradyarrhythmias

Bradycardia occurs as either a primary cardiac event or secondary to other noncardiac occurrences. The primary cardiac causes include congenital complete heart block, sick sinus syndrome (seen frequently after the Mustard procedure for D-transposition of the great arteries or after Fontan operation). Secondary causes are hypoxia, acidosis, electrolyte abnormalities (hypoglycemia, hypocalcemia, etc.), drug overdose, etc. Accurate diagnosis requires a rhythm strip from multiple leads and, at times, an atrial recording via either the transesophageal route or through temporary epicardial pacing wires. Treatment for the cardiac causes include atropine (0.02 mg/kg per dose with a minimum dose of 0.1 mg), isoproterenol infusion (0.02 to 0.1 mg/kg per minute), epinephrine (0.01 mg/kg) or temporary pacing via a transesophageal pacing catheter, epicardial pacing wires, transvenous pacing catheter, or external transthoracic patches. For noncardiac etiologies, correction of the underlying cause is necessary.

Tachyarrhythmias

Sinus tachycardia is the most common cause of a tachyarrhythmia and is caused by decreased cardiac output, anemia, hypovolemia, pain, catecholamines, fever, etc. Correcting the underlying problem resolves the tachyarrhythmia. When tachyarrhythmias are not sinus in origin, they are caused by either reentry or automatic foci arising from any level of the conduction system, such as the sinus node, atrium, atrioventricular node, His bundle, Purkinje system, and ventricle. Following is a discussion of the common types of tachyarrhythmias found in children.

Supraventricular Tachycardia. Supraventricular tachycardia (SVT) is any tachycardia arising from above the His bundle. and is commonly narrow complex (QRS less than 0.12 ms or 0.10 ms in neonates). Rarely, it is wide complex because of a bundle branch block or antedromic conduction.

Wolff Parkinson White Syndrome (WPW). WPW is diagnosed by a short PR interval (less than 0.10 ms) with the presence of a delta wave (slurring of the initial portion of the QRS complex) on the surface ECG while in sinus rhythm. In the tachyarrhythmia, the QRS complex is usually narrow and rarely wide. The tachyarrhythmia is the result of a circus movement. Typically, there is slow conduction from the atrium through the AV node with rapid retrograde conduction through the accessory connection (Bundle of Kent) from the ventricle back into the atrium thus completing the circuit. This is called orthodromic tachycardia. Antedromic tachycardia occurs when the impulse is transmitted from the atria directly to the ventricle through the accessory connection with subsequent retrograde conduction through the AV node back into the atrium. This results in a wide complex tachycardia and is significantly more life-threatening because ventricular fibrillation can occur. Acute treatment involves synchronized DC cardioversion for any patient who is unstable (shock, hypotension, arrest, etc.) at a dose of 0.5 to 2 J/kg. If the patient is stable, vagal maneuvers can be tried typically with only fair success. Adenosine has become the drug of choice for the treatment of acute SVT in a hemodynamically stable patient. An intravenous dose of 50 to 250 μg/kg is RAPIDLY infused causing a brief episode of bradycardia lasting a few seconds. Atropine should be available at the bedside along with the full cadre of resuscitation equipment. Propranolol, esmolol, verapamil (ONLY in children more than 1 year), procainamide, quinidine, flecainide, and amiodarone have all been used to treat this arrhythmia. Transesophageal or temporary epicardial overdrive pacing can also be used to convert a patient from SVT to sinus rhythm when the arrhythmia is caused by a reentry phenomenon.

Concealed Accessory Connections. SVT can occur through other accessory connections that have slow conduction properties resulting in an identical set of conditions to that in WPW, but without the slurring of the QRS or antedromic tachycardia. These patients are at less risk of sudden death. Treatment is as described for patients with WPW.

Atrial Tachycardia. Atrial tachycardia occurs as the result of either reentry (atrial flutter), atrial automaticity, or atrial fibrillation.

Atrial Flutter. Atrial flutter occurs as the result of reentry within the atrium. Diagnostic flutter waves can be seen on surface ECG. Treatment centers on controlling atrio-ventricular conduction by causing block in the AV node. This can be accomplished by using many agents including: digoxin, esmolol, propranolol, procainamide, quinidine, and amiodarone. Overdrive pacing can also be effective. Conversion of the flutter to sinus rhythm is accomplished by a variety of means, including antiarrhythmia medications, overdrive pacing, and DC synchronized cardioversion.

Atrial Ectopic Tachycardia (AET). AET arises from a small abnormal focus of tissue within the atrium. Typically this rhythm increases slowly to its highest rate ("warms up") and decreases slowly back to sinus rhythm ("slows down"). Vagal maneuvers, adenosine, and overdrive pacing are ineffective at converting this arrhythmia. It is refractory to most antiarrhythmic agents, but can be successfully treated with radiofrequency ablation or cryoablation techniques.

Atrial Fibrillation. Atrial fibrillation results in an irregular rhythm with variable ventricular conduction. Initial treatment is focused on controlling AV conduction then secondarily converting atrial fibrillation into sinus rhythm. Before converting patients, one must exclude any atrial thrombus by echocardiography. If a thrombus is present and patients are converted to sinus rhythm, the thrombus may embolize. Anticoagulation must be performed in this setting. Treatment is similar to that for atrial flutter. Patients may only respond to DC cardioversion and overdrive pacing is usually ineffective.

Accelerated Junctional Ectopic Tachycardia (JET). JET is a common and lethal arrhythmia found in the CTICU that historically results in death in 50% of children. The diagnosis of JET is made when a narrow complex tachycardia occurs with AV dissociation in a postoperative patient. Initial supportive measures involve correcting any electrolyte (sodium, potassium, calcium, phosphate, magnesium, and glucose) or blood-gas abnormalities (acidemia, hypercapnia, hypoxemia), transfusing red blood cells for anemia to optimize cardiac output and oxygen delivery, and controlling fever and pain. Excessive catecholamine infusions should be decreased, but is seldom possible because most children are in cardiogenic shock. Cooling of individuals helps decrease the rate of JET, but must be done after paralysis and deep-pain control to prevent shivering and discomfort. Once the ventricular rate is slowed, AV sequential pacing should be initiated to improve cardiac output. Many antiarrhythmic agents have been used to attempt to control the arrhythmia with only a few being successful. The most useful agents are amiodarone (5 mg/kg slow intravenous load followed by an infusion of 5 μg/kg per minute) and propafenone (100 mg/m^2 per day PO for 3 days). Rarely, radiofrequency ablation is necessary to create complete AV block. Improved survival can be accomplished with meticulous CTICU care combined with the previously noted therapies and time for the patients to recover from their surgical procedures.

Ventricular Arrhythmias

Premature Ventricular Contractions (PVCs). Isolated, unifocal PVCs are found frequently in normal children and adolescents. In the CTICU, PVCs should be assumed to be pathologic and then determined to be benign. Multifocal or coupled PVCs are an ominous finding. Electrolyte abnormalities (sodium, potassium, calcium, phosphate, magnesium, and glucose) or blood-gas abnormalities (acidemia, hypercapnia, hypoxemia) are the most common causes of PVCs. These derangements should be sought and corrected. Central venous monitoring lines should not be placed within the ventricular cavity. Drug-induced ventricular arrhythmias should be excluded (i.e., digoxin). In the immediate postoperative patient, PVCs may be the first indicator of myocardial ischemia. If so, myocardial oxygen delivery should be improved and myocardial oxygen consumption should be decreased. Excessive use of catecholamines can cause PVCs. If treatment is necessary, lidocaine, β-blockers, and dilantin are effective at suppressing PVCs.

Ventricular Tachycardia. Ventricular tachycardia occurs with regularity in the CTICU. In unstable patients, synchronized DC cardioversion at a dose of 2 to 4 J/kg is given. One must be prepared for the arrhythmia to degenerate to ventricular fibrillation. In stable patients, lidocaine can be given as a bolus (1 mg/kg) followed by infusion at a rate of 10 to 50 μg/kg per minute. Other agents successful in treating ventricular tachycardia include propranolol, flecainide, propafenone, and amiodarone.

Torsades de Pointes. Torsades de Pointes is polymorphic ventricular tachycardia that can occur in children with idiopathic Long QT syndrome or acquired Long QT syndrome from electrolyte abnormalities (hypocalcemia, hypomagnesemia) or medications (quinidine, procainamide, disopyramide, tricyclic antidepressants, phenothiazines, cisapride). The approach to treatment of these patients is multifaceted. Asynchronous defibrillation is used in any hemodynamically unstable patient. Lidocaine infusion may or may not be of benefit. β-blockade is effective for treating this arrhythmia in children with idiopathic Long QT syndrome. Magnesium sulfate bolus infusion (50 mg/kg) can terminate torsades de pointes. Any electrolyte abnormality should be corrected and any QT-lengthening drug should be discontinued. Atrial pacing is used to prevent the increased prolongation of the QT interval that occurs with bradycardia.

Ventricular Fibrillation. Ventricular fibrillation is cardiac standstill resulting from the uncoordinated depolarization of the myocardium. It is an ominous rhythm with fatal results. Treatment involves initiation of CPR, asynchronous defibrillation with 2 J/kg of energy then 4 J/kg and this dose is repeated if no resolution occurs. Epinephrine (0.01 mg/kg) is given followed by attempted cardioversion. Lidocaine (1 mg/kg) is then given and cardioversion attempted again. Bretylium is given (5 mg/kg) with attempted cardioversion. Finally, a third dose of lidocaine or bretylium is given followed by cardioversion.

Cardiac Pacing

Standard terminology for pacing involves a three-letter abbreviation (in its simplest form). The first letter stands for where pacing is occurring with options being A, atrial; V, ventricle; and D, dual (both atrium and ventricle). The second letter stands for where sensing occurs with options being A, atrial; V, ventricle; D, dual (either atrium and ventricle); and O, no sensing. The third letter stands for the action of the pacemaker when there is a sensed event with options being I, inhibit pacemaker output when a sensed event occurs; T, trigger pacemaker when sensed event occurs; D, dual (both inhibit or trigger when sensed event occurs); O, no response. Common pacing modes would be VVI, which stands for pacing the ventricle, and if an event (ventricular depolarization) is sensed, inhibit output from the pacemaker to the ventricle to prevent a Q-wave-on-T-wave event that could result in ventricular fibrillation. This mode commonly is used for surgical complete AV block. A pacemaker in AAI mode would pace the atrium, and if an event (atrial depolarization) is sensed, inhibit output from the pacemaker to the atrium to prevent a premature atrial contraction. This mode is used commonly for sinus bradycardia. A pacemaker in DDD mode would pace both the atrium and ventricle, and if an event (atrial or ventricular depolarization) is sensed, inhibit or trigger output from the pacemaker to the atrium or ventricle. Although this mode is significantly more complex than others, it allows for normal AV conduction and is the preferred mode for temporary pacing.

Fluid Management

The fluid management for all patients in the CTICU must be precisely managed. Many patients with congestive heart failure and most postoperative patients must be fluid-restricted (0.5 to 0.75 × maintenance fluids). Particularly in small infants, the infusion of glucose must be more than 6 to 8 mg/kg per minute in order to prevent hypoglycemia. Frequent bedside glucose checks must be performed. Once patients are beyond the immediate postoperative period, fluid should be liberalized and calories increased. Diuretics are used to assist in maximizing caloric intake and maintain fluid balance. Electrolytes (sodium, potassium, chloride, urea nitrogen, creatinine, calcium, and magnesium) must be monitored frequently, particularly during rapid diuresis.

Transfusion Medicine

Oxygen-carrying capacity must be maximized for children with cardiac disease. Hematocrits should be checked frequently in patients with CHD. No absolute numbers can be given for a minimum hematocrit necessary for patients with CHD. The following is meant as a GENERAL GUIDELINE. For asymptomatic patients with insignificant disease (i.e., mild pulmonary stenosis), a hematocrit of more than 20% is acceptable. For patients with acyanotic heart disease with mild symptoms (i.e., moderate size VSD), a hematocrit of more than 30% is acceptable. For patients with acyanotic heart disease with significant symptoms (i.e., large size VSD with CHF), a hematocrit of more than 35% is necessary. For mildly cyanotic patients (i.e., SaO_2 more than 90%), a hematocrit of more than 35% is acceptable. For moderately cyanotic patients (i.e., SaO_2 75 to 80%), a hematocrit of more than 40% is necessary. Packed red blood cells are the most common product transfused for this purpose.

Platelets are consumed and made dysfunctional by the cardiopulmonary bypass machine. Even if the platelet count is normal, platelets should be transfused in the bleeding postoperative patient. Fresh, frozen plasma is transfused for bleeding patients with an elevated prothrombin and/or activated partial thromboplastin time. Cryoprecipitate has high concentrations of Von Willebrand's Factor and fibrinogen and can be transfused in patients with hypofibrinogenemia.

Several pharmacologic agents may help control bleeding in children after congenital heart surgery. Protamine is given in the operating room to reverse the effects of heparin, which is necessary to place the patient on cardiopulmonary bypass. A repeat dose may be necessary in the CTICU. Aprotinin is a serine protease inhibitor that affects platelet function, the intrinsic pathway of coagulation, and fibrinolysis. Aprotinin decreases bleeding in adults after bypass surgery; however, there are mixed results in children. ϵ–Aminocaproic acid, an inhibitor of the fibrinolysis, helps control postoperative bleeding in children.

Index

Page numbers in *italics* denote figures; those followed by "t" denote tables.